1998

The
New
Rules of
Healthcare
Marketing
23 strategies for success

The New Rules of Healthcare Marketing

23 strategies for success

Arthur C. Sturm, Jr.

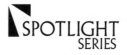

SPOTLIGHT
SERIES

Health Administration Press

02 01 00 99 98   5 4 3 2 1

Library of Congress Cataloging-in-Publication Data

The new rules of healthcare marketing : 23 strategies for success / by Arthur C. Sturm, Jr.
    p. cm.
Includes bibliographical references.
ISBN 1-56793-074-3
1. Medical care—Marketing.   2. Integrated delivery of healthcare.
I. Title.
RA410.56.S78   1998
362.1'068'8—dc21   97-42425
                                                                    CIP

Health Administration Press
A division of the Foundation
of the American College of Healthcare Executives
One North Franklin
Suite 1700
Chicago, IL 60606
312/424–2800

This book is dedicated to the crew members of *ChristoLee* for their ability to keep me on a true course, their support through storms and sunshine, and their stunning lesson that life is a real trip.

Table of Contents

Acknowledgments

Writing is never a solo activity. Invention and creativity need the hard facts of research, the observations of respected peers, and the continuing support of friends and family.

Among those who had the patience and courage to work with me are the following, to whom I owe my gratitude: the staff at Find/SVP; Liz Medina; John Eudes; my partners, Rob Rosenberg and Donna King; people sitting next to me on late-night flights (sorry about the loud keyboard work); my clients for the opportunity to work with them; Tom Atchison; Kathleen Harkness; technology that allowed me to work anywhere, anytime. I am grateful, too, for the persistence of change that continues to influence all of our daily lives.

Fundamentals

The new rules of healthcare marketing are based on three very simple ideas: the brand, relationships, and results. They are inextricably linked. Everything you do should relate to these three drivers.

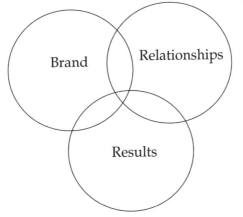

The brand: A brand is the summation of all the elements of your organization—from what it offers to how it performs to what it promises. The brand is the overarching promise that is made to the market and must be fulfilled every time you create a transaction.

Relationships: Healthcare, perhaps more than any other business in America, is about relationships. The most fundamental relationship is the one between doctor and patient. But the successful IDN must create relationships that allow it to enhance and support that core strategy. It's not about customers; it's about creating emotional, physical, and financial bonds that last.

Results: Without them, you're dead.

Introduction

As we all know by now, the "rules of the game" in healthcare are changing. Hospitals, physician practices, and other entities are teaming up to work with a daunting alphabet soup of arrangements, from IDNs (integrated delivery networks) to GPWWs (group practices without walls) to OWAs (other weird arrangements). Competitors are becoming collaborators, not-for-profit organizations are becoming for-profit holding companies, and so on and so on. Under the influence of managed care, hospitals appear to be on the verge of becoming just another commodity, giving up their role as the unchallenged center of the healthcare universe. This is raising intensified competition among providers and among managed care plans—it's giving purchasers and consumers more and more leverage in demanding broader access, improved service, and greater accountability through outcomes reporting.

With all of this change, where does healthcare marketing fit? Right in the middle of things! The targets have changed, the strategies have changed, and so have the tactics. So it becomes overwhelmingly obvious that the basic rules of healthcare marketing must change, too.

More than ever the right marketing is essential in a healthcare organization's ability to navigate the uncharted waters of a changing environment. Marketing is intertwined with vision, organizational culture, strategic planning, and program development. Marketing is a way for your organization to focus its efforts and sustain that focus. Marketing is a way for your staff's skills, talent, and dedication to reach out and help your community. And, I might add, marketing is basic to your very survival in a competitive marketplace.

The overarching goal of this book is to provide an engaging refresher to healthcare marketing. The book is not a treatise. Although faculty and students in health administration may well find the book useful, it does not have a traditional academic tone. Neither is it an exhaustive how-to book. The healthcare executives who form the target audience probably will delegate the nitty-gritty details about marketing to staff or consultants. This book does, however, link several goals:

- **To demystify marketing.** The book seeks to answer basic questions like these: What role does marketing play in the new environment? How can marketing help drive our mission and strategies?

- **To explain what marketing has to do with success in today's environment.** The book explains the lively role that marketing needs to play in an era of managed care, integration, and intense competition.

- **To provide a reference source.** By dividing the book into short chapters, each covering a specific marketing "rule," the book should provide easy reference for all readers. Want to start a team working on brand identity? A good way to begin might be to read Rule 3, "Your Brand Is a Valuable Asset: Nurture and Develop It," for an explanation of the concept of brand identity.

- **To entertain.** The book is written in a conversational style; it even attempts some humor. It is short enough to read on a plane ride and should be engaging enough to keep you awake. You might even find a chuckle or two after a long day of tedious meetings.

• **To inspire.** The book should leave you with a renewed sense of your goals as a healthcare executive—and the feeling that you actually *can* meet those goals.

For healthcare executives, trustees, physicians, and other professionals interested in the business side of healthcare, this book should be a pleasurable, enlightening reintroduction to marketing . . . and a tool for success in the vastly important pursuit of providing healthcare to your community.

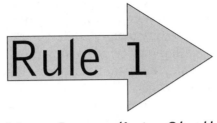

Rule 1

Your Immediate Challenge Is to Move from Promise to Proof

Integrated delivery networks (IDNs), much like other marvels of modern medicine, are making some rather substantial promises to the marketplace. Basically, they say that the acquisition of physician practices, the development of broad geographic networks, and other business efforts will result in lower costs and better care.

The equation is familiar to most businesses. They, too, have done their share of consolidating, reorganizing, and the like. But more and more, healthcare executives and consumers are asking for some evidence that this disruption in healthcare will deliver the promised results.

Let's look at some of the promises and at where in general IDNs seem to be in relation to those promises. Marketing will be key both in helping an IDN focus on how to fulfill the promises and in helping communicate the network's achievements to the community.

Lower Costs

Who can argue with the need to lower the cost of anything? However, for the IDN, the cost message is a difficult one to send successfully. Price becomes the reason to buy in the absence of a more compelling argument. In the consumer market, price wars have demonstrated that marketshare shifts to the company with the price promotion only while the price promotion is in play. Drop the discount and the share returns to pre-promotion levels.

Research has shown that cost messages for healthcare consumers represent a double-edged sword. On the one hand, consumers are glad to hear that the price has gone down; on the other, they fear that the cost reduction is at the expense of quality. Given the relatively little experience consumers have with healthcare costs in general, the claim of lower costs is somewhat difficult for them to grasp. "Lower" implies that consumers know the average. But as we all know, they don't. So if you run out with strictly a "lower cost" message, you may be positioning your brand somewhat unfavorably from the start. Make sure that the cost is where you want it to be, because repositioning yourself out of that niche in the future will be hard to do.

Retailer Wal-Mart will own the low-price position in perpetuity. No promotion on the face of the earth is going to convince consumers to think otherwise.

Greater Clinical Firepower

This is the dream promise. Saying that "we've amassed this well-integrated regional medical staff that now is sharing best practices" is a somewhat questionable claim. Clinical firepower—the ability to truly integrate a clinical offering—should and must be the goal of the IDN. It represents the best way to reach the goal of highest possible quality at the most reasonable cost. In most markets, and for newly formed IDNs, it's a message of the future.

Easier Access

This claim has always mystified me. Access to what? Basic care? That's an economic issue, and unless the IDN is funding indigent care there is no "easier access."

Access to a broader range of specialists? Conceptually and potentially, yes. But as a practical matter it's a tenuous claim. Yes, you can say your physician referral service has more specialists who are more broadly distributed, but since you haven't measurably changed the *actual* supply or quality, there really isn't much to say beyond that.

Greater Community Involvement

Here's a vastly unexplored idea of some, although limited, potential. Just about every provider has done a community-needs assessment. And just about all of the assessments, at least in urban areas, show that America's households are swimming in stress—stress so great that it often leads to domestic violence, increased use of alcohol and drugs, depression or other mental health problems, or some such combination.

Historically, social pathologies fall into clinical areas that have not been of primary interest to hospitals. They don't necessarily fall into neat, established clinical categories. And they don't fill beds. But in an industry without heroes, the institution that takes the higher ground and advocates the common good may find many rewards. More on this topic later.

Fulfilling the Promises

Three broad ideas for moving from promise to proof are worth considering for healthcare executives. One is based on

General Electric's popular slogan, another I call "the navigator," and a third on "emerging." All are ideas for positioning an IDN's vast array of services in terms of customer benefit.

"We bring good things to life"

Years ago General Electric began to use this slogan to illustrate how the company aggregated a number of diverse products into a single benefit for the consumer. It used the simple but convincing tag line: "We bring good things to life." It was a marvelous way for a diversified products company to position itself favorably across several lines of business. It spoke of benefit. It had emotion. And it somehow convinced us that a company that made appliances, jet engines, and nuclear reactors was a good, friendly company.

Perhaps there is a similar position for IDNs. Currently they appear to be thinking on a rather linear plane, referencing so many of these properties and so many of those programs. While reviewing your capabilities helps an audience understand how and where your products fit into their lives, a broader, more conceptual approach might be fresher and more effective. An IDN doesn't need to be defined by its properties, but by its abilities. One way is to, well, bring good things to life.

The Navigator

As IDNs mature to the point where they can talk about their integrated staffs and programs, there is another role they can play that is clearly needed by the community and beneficial to the organization. It's what I call the *navigator strategy.*

Hospitals have had some experience with this type of strategy by using their telemarketing services as a means to register people for programs, direct physician referrals, and distribute health education information. While these services answer ongoing personal consumer needs, an IDN can harness that same technology more broadly, providing information and aid to the community in general, and subsequently gaining direct referrals not just to its physicians but to all of its business entities.

The "Emerging" Solution

Somehow, many marketers have come to the conclusion that the promise of an IDN has to be something that's totally accomplished. If that's the case, it's going to be years before some systems can utter their first word.

Perhaps one strategy worth pursuing is similar to that of United Airlines (UAL). Through what looks like some very smart research, UAL discovered that their target, the business traveler, viewed most airline advertising as a bunch of baloney. And they probably also discovered that even their most loyal users found their service plan to be more of a burden than a help.

United took a big risk. It decided to address those concerns head-on in their advertising by admitting that business travel is a hassle and that they are working to make things better. Thus the "United rising" campaign was born. It's a gutsy, risky strategy that makes a major promise that things are going to change. Food. Service. Equipment. They're all being reviewed and redone.

That's certainly a welcome message, but it begs a cynical response.

Perhaps the same acknowledgment would work well for an IDN. The promise is one of change to come, not so much one of change that's happened. It is in many ways marketing the vision of IDNs rather than their accomplishments.

As much as I favor this type of approach, you must remember that it creates expectations. And the expectations are probably pretty substantial. United raised my expectations. They told me food in coach class would improve. So imagine my reaction to the flight that not only served the same stale sandwich as before, but ran commercials during the in-flight movie telling me how things were going to change. The first time I saw that ad, I laughed. The second time, I knew that their promise was a joke.

As we will review later, promises in large service organizations are difficult to deliver. In the absence of a more substantive argument, marketing the vision could be successful, but sooner or later, you'll still have to deliver.

It is clear from a number of consumer studies that the general public feels confused—cast adrift in its search for health solutions. An IDN by definition is supposed to have many of those solutions within its organization. By positioning itself as a resource for solutions to health problems, rather than as a collection of physical facilities, it may provide a greater community benefit.

Admittedly such a strategy could create an avalanche of phone calls, and you'll need to put steps in place to manage the demand. But such a structure seems within reach, and the strategy is worth considering.

What promises did your IDN make to the communities it serves? Chances are they were many. And there is equal probability that patience is wearing thin. It's time to deliver.

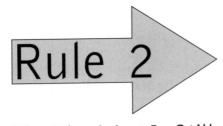

Rule 2

The Physician Is Still the Focal Point of the Relationship

While the "new healthcare" may be changing the physician's roles, exchanging the physician's powers, and otherwise reinventing the physician, one constant remains. To most Americans, healthcare is defined as their relationship with their physician. And while staff models and other forms of assembly line care have attempted to change that relationship, the focus, for many, remains on the physician.

Marketers must also remember that IDNs and their properties are usually faceless organizations. They talk about all they can do for people, but unless they put a "someone human" in the equation, it's a pretty flat discussion.

Research continues to reinforce the fact that consumers are struggling with the notion of an integrated delivery system. Try as we might to explain it, they still just don't get it. But they seem to have a clear understanding of "their physician" and his or her role in their life. We should listen to that finding and act accordingly. Until the IDN becomes more tangible, more meaningful to consumers, the physician will continue to be the focus of their perceptions of healthcare. And even if the industry is successful in creating a clear perception of an IDN, the physician may still be the central figure.

The Physician as the Brand

Is an IDN defined by its medical staff? Today it can be. The challenge to the marketer is to find creative ways to distinguish the skills and credentials of that medical staff from those of the competition.

A physician-based strategy will succeed with only one IDN in each market. And that's the IDN that gets the message there first. A second entry into the market with the same position cannot succeed.

Why? It goes to what marketing gurus Al Ries and Jack Trout call the immutable "Law of Leadership." In this scenario, Trout and Ries state that whoever gets to the market first becomes the leader and owns the position. They cite examples of Federal Express, Tylenol, and even American air hero Charles Lindbergh. Each of those brands has become so dominant in its respective category that it is often difficult to identify just who is in second place.

The same opportunity is available to one and only one IDN in each market.

If Not the Brand, Then the Endorser

Our work with integrated networks shows increasing resistance by physician groups to be "branded" by the new parent. Even though these physicians are technically network employees, they insist on a separate branded presence.

If you're stymied in your effort to use physicians as your brand, maybe there's a better way to make them part of your total effort. And that's by having the physicians become endorsers of the integration strategy.

An endorser's effort plays quite simply. There, physicians talk to the marketplace about the benefits of integration. The idea: "See what I can do now that I'm part of a system. I have greater access to research, to tertiary care, to other physician expertise." That's a little dispassionate, but the idea is there. The physician is not a spokesperson, but someone who communicates the benefit of the system by talking about a true benefit to the consumer.

Obviously the strategy can be played out with any number of healthcare professionals. Nurses, home care workers, and others can talk in practical terms about the advantages of being part of a system.

Admittedly, the emerging system may have to talk about "work in progress," meaning that some of the benefits are still coming into place. But that's a far better approach than not using physicians at all.

Executing a physician strategy for an IDN can be extremely tricky and loaded with political land mines. But the course can be navigated, and the trip may well be worth taking.

In a May 28, 1997, article in the *Wall Street Journal,* a report on Columbia/HCA Healthcare Corp (Nashville, Tennessee) suggested that the company sees a diminished role for the physician in the not-too-distant future. Other clinicians would take the physician's place. Perhaps that will occur. But until that time, Americans will continue to define healthcare as their relationship with their physician. It's likely to take a generation of change to unravel that bond.

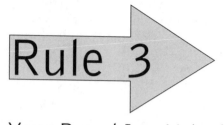

Rule 3

Your Brand Is a Valuable Asset: Nurture and Develop It

One of a provider's greatest assets never appears on its balance sheet. It's called "brand equity." Put simply, this phrase means that the reputation an organization enjoys in the market is a true asset it can leverage to your advantage to increase membership, redirect marketshare, and pave the way for other opportunities.

But having and nurturing a brand are different from simply promoting one.

A brand is the sum of the experiences the consumer has with the product. The price, the performance, the satisfaction of the product are what make it unique and appealing. Too often healthcare providers equate image with brand, but a single ingredient such as that has never built or sustained a lasting brand.

If image were all there is to branding, marketing would be a relatively simple task. Marketers could whip up some advertising, make some outrageous claims, and *voila*, it's a brand. Of course it doesn't work that way. Branding is a conscious and ongoing effort. You have to decide what you want your brand to be and then deliver on that promise to your customers.

The challenge today, particularly for emerging integrated systems, is to make a true brand out of their collection of acquired facilities, physicians, and employees. And at the core of that challenge is the need for consistency. Brands thrive on consistency. It's that day-in, day-out performance that creates the brand. A brand delivers on a promise it makes to the consumer day after day after day. It sounds pretty dull and boring, but managing the performance of a brand to meet customer expectations over and over again is no small task. And in a highly diversified environment such as healthcare networks, the challenge is exponentially greater.

Choosing a Brand Model

Many CEOs of IDNs have told me of the difficulty they're having in applying the notion of a brand to their organization. As an aid, my partners and I developed an exercise that uses several major international companies as brand models. The goal is to see if any of these existing brand models can be applied to a specific IDN. There is no right or wrong answer: it is an exercise in creativity and strategy.

The companies we chose were General Electric (GE), BASF, Procter & Gamble (P&G), and Nabisco. Each represents a different approach to branding that may or may not be translatable to healthcare.

To populate the example here, we'll use a fictitious "ABC Health System" as an example.

General Electric

General Electric of Fairfield, Connecticut, is a multinational manufacturer of consumer and industrial products. It is highly diversified, but has chosen to build one brand around a central theme: "We bring good things to life" (which I've always thought would be the ideal tag line for a healthcare organization).

The characteristics of this brand strategy:

- Products are not independently branded.
- The "GE" name appears on every product.
- The company is positioned as "making life better" through all of its products.
- Advertising supports the brand and products across multiple industries.
- A strong emotional connection is created across its various markets.

The healthcare translation, or, ABC the GE way:

- ABC is the brand.
- ABC brand replaces the names of the organization's other entities
  Example: from North Community Hospital to ABC Hospital/North County
- Advertising focuses on the positive role ABC plays in people's lives.
- The ABC brand crosses all markets: consumer, purchaser, professional.

Why would you want to consider using this strategy?

It's very much a global position that shows the diversity of the organization and the many ways it serves the community. The main take-away is that this is a company with good products and I (the consumer) should probably trust these people. It's really more of an awareness campaign than it is positioning. GE's national telemarketing center is a critical link in this strategy allowing the company to create a relationship and provide product information across all of its consumer lines. If you can change the name of the facilities, and you're still struggling with a definitive position, a softer approach like GE's might work well.

BASF

This multinational chemical company based in Ludwigshafen, Germany, doesn't have any branded products. In fact, that was the marketing challenge it faced. BASF wanted the market to know that it was an essential part of products (e.g., the "Intel inside" idea), but it didn't want the market to know about its specific products. Thus the tag line: "We don't make a lot of the products you buy. We make a lot of the products you buy better." We called this the "enabler" strategy, meaning that their products help other products be better.

Thus, the BASF strategy:

- The brand strategy supports a corporation, not a product.
- Products are not identified by brand names; other people's products benefit from them.
- Advertising demonstrates product attributes.

. . . ABC the BASF way:

- ABC is the branded entity.
- Products may or may not be independently branded; individual branding is not critical to the success of the strategy.
- Products become secondary to the value of the overall brand.
- The brand is positioned as "being behind making your physicians and hospitals better."
- A demonstration of the value of the brand is its ability to strengthen local programs (e.g., "This innovation at Community Hospital—brought to you by ABC").

Why consider this strategy?

The BASF model is for those organizations that want to articulate the role of an overall IDN. As a holding company, an IDN has a hard time communicating its benefit. By showing that it is the *source* of improving healthcare in the community, the holding company now has meaning. There is an unresolved question of balance; that is, in this scenario should you weigh the effort totally at the corporate entity or in a mix with the business units? That's more a judgment call than a question with an answer. Your individual business situation will determine which way is best.

Procter & Gamble

Procter & Gamble of Cincinnati, Ohio, is a world leader in the manufacturing and marketing of consumer products. A major part of its strategy is to own a category rather than just a share of it. For example, P&G markets several brands of coffee that clearly compete against each other. P&G encourages that competition to build both the brands and the category resulting in a larger category share for P&G.

The strategy:

- Brand strategy is developed at the product level with little to no corporate visibility (Folgers Coffee versus Hills Brothers).
- Products each have a unique position and brand personality with different target audiences.
- Corporate leverage occurs at the wholesale level (distribution, advertising).
- Brand managers fight for corporate resources but share philosophies and goals.

  . . . ABC the P&G way:

- Brand strategy centers on each ABC unit: Children's Hospital, North Community Hospital, and so on.

- ABC is seen as a "good citizen"—not as the brand.
- ABC negotiates at the wholesale level (managed care contracts) while its brands operate at the retail level (physician practices, hospitals, etc).

Why use this strategy?

Originally, this strategy was not favored much in the health-care market. But the more I think about it, the more applicable it is to many markets. As consolidation continues, large, well-preferred brands will face the possibility of being consumed by other large, well-preferred brands. Should all of that brand equity be abandoned under a consolidated name? Maybe that's not such a good idea. Maybe those individual brands should survive—and in fact compete against each other—on the retail level, while broader strategies are created at the wholesale level.

Nabisco

Nabisco of Parsippany, New Jersey, manufactures and markets a wide range of food products from salty snacks to confectioneries. The company brands each product independently, but uses the Nabisco name as a seal of quality, an assurance that SnackWell products, for example, are something you would like because they were created by a quality company.

The strategy:

- Focus is on individual brands with individual features and benefits.
- The parent brand is positioned as a quality company; it creates an overall halo.
  (Note the use of a musical tag on radio and TV in the form of the single word "Na-bis-co.")

- The parent identification is apparent on each package, but not dominant.
- Sales promotion crosses multiple product lines.

. . . ABC the Nabisco way

- Each entity is the branded product.
- ABC is in "the backdrop." Not dominant.
- Promotion is independently pursued among entities.
- Contracting is done at the wholesale level, sales at the retail level.

Why consider this strategy?

The Nabisco platform is very much a hybrid of GE and P&G. It works because Nabisco has spent years developing credibility for its name while marketing products that reinforce the parent's commitment to quality. Its flaw for healthcare, if there is one, is twofold. First, it requires time to build the reputation of the parent and, second, it requires strong financial support for each of the independent brands.

Which of these models, if any, is appropriate to your organization will be a subject of considerable internal discussion, market research, and painful thinking. As I say throughout this book, choose wisely.

The Brand's Infrastructure: Positioning

Marketing a brand has two basic "infrastructure" elements: its unique features and its positioning in the market. You can't have one without the other.

There are many elements to a brand, but often they can be shared by many competitors. As mentioned, quality of the medical staff can be shared, as can things like broad geographic distribution, available tertiary services, and other attributes. To differentiate your brand, you must position it effectively in the market.

"Positioning" is deciding where and how you want your brand to fit in the market. A little further on, we'll talk about the elements that constitute the Marriott Hotels's position. But when you look at the elements, you'll be able to say that they could be shared by any brand. It's how Marriott has worked to uniquely own those attributes that set it apart.

A Positioning Exercise

There is a handy fill-in-the-blanks exercise IDNs may want to use in developing their positioning. It's as old as the hills, as they say—and for a reason. It works.

The equation looks like this:

> To (our Target Audiences) NewCo is a (Frame of Reference) that has/does (Point of Difference) because (Reason to Believe).

Let's dissect this equation.

Target Audience

It's important to understand up front just who it is you want to receive your attention. Is it payors? Physicians? Consumers? Employees? Stakeholders? Legislators?

It's okay to have more than one target audience, but you may find it difficult to position yourself to multiple audiences in one positioning statement. Thus you can write different positioning statements for each audience, but obviously you have to find a thread that weaves things together. Lack of commonality is disasterous for a brand. Without it your brand will unravel.

You may also decide that you have primary and secondary targets. There's nothing wrong with that either. This exercise helps you sort out that issue as well.

Frame of Reference

This determination is particularly critical for IDNs. Frame of reference speaks to the kind of companies with which you want to be compared. For example, General Motors wants to be compared with domestic transportation manufacturers; Merck with global pharmaceutical companies, and so on.

IDNs are challenged to find a frame of reference. There is no existing category called "integrated delivery networks," and the old standby of regional hospital organization is way too limiting. IDNs are breaking new ground and have to find a familiar concept (or a concept that can be self-defining) to which their audiences can link themselves. People like to buy the familiar. If you are a new category of services, there will be initial resistance. Time, consistency, and exposure will overcome the resistance, but you still have to do business while the market catches up.

One option is to choose a broad category like "regional service company" or to create something new such as "community benefit organization." True, finding your frame of reference is a huge challenge, but it's critical to the development of your strategy and the execution of your basic mission.

Research among your targets is essential to identify what your market can grasp or "permit" you to pursue. Positioning must be single-minded—one position *only* for each player in a category. If one system owns the position of leadership in specialty care, then they alone own it. But they can't own specialty care, convenience, *and* best overall care. Our minds don't have that many compartments to put them in. Someone else in the market can own what others don't.

Point of Difference

This factor is exactly what it says it is: the singular thing for which you want the market to recognize you. Sounds simple enough, but the degree of difficulty increases exponentially as you try to whittle down the long list of possibilities to one idea. Note the number of ideas you can have—one. Only one. Being all things to all people is not a position, it's chaos. Brands in chaos don't make it.

To add to the complexity of the analysis, your point of difference has to be "available," meaning that your competitor hasn't already seized it. FedEx debuted as an express delivery service (its frame of reference) that delivered packages by noon the next day (its point of difference). Now it's pretty clear that any company in the express delivery service can get a package to its destination by noon the next day, but FedEx discovered that no one was exploiting that position. It seized it, spent to own it, and became the invincible leader in the category.

In theory, IDNs can share points of difference but whoever gets to the market first and spends to own the position is the winner. Who's in second place in overnight delivery? Who knows? And, frankly, no one cares.

Reason to Believe

It's just what it says it is. A reason to believe. In FedEx's case, the market believed what it said because delivery was guaranteed "absolutely, positively."

There is no positioning statement without a reason to believe.

So, let's run out the FedEx positioning statement as I've constructed it, with all due apologies to FedEx:

> To *individuals responsible for priority shipments*, FedEx is the *express delivery company* that *will have your package delivered by noon the next day* because *it has a money-back guarantee*.

Providers need to take a hard look at their reason to believe. It's the part of the statement that is most often ignored. If you leave out the reason to believe, you essentially have little more than a boastful claim. Example:

> *"We are the leaders in cardiology."* . . . That's pretty empty. *"We are leaders in cardiology because we have the best-trained physicians in the region."* . . . Now *there's* a reason to believe.

A Look at a Service Brand

Let's look at an example from another industry to illustrate the point.

Most of my professional life is spent traveling. One thing that we road warriors do to reduce stress is eliminate as many surprises as possible. So we tend to give our business consistently to those travel partners who we believe will give us the fewest surprises. Note that we are not necessarily looking for partners who will exceed our expectations, but for those who will perform in an *expected* manner at an *anticipated* price across a *wide geographical* range. If those criteria sound familiar, good. In many ways they reflect those of an IDN.

To illustrate my point, I'll talk about hotels. When I travel, I prefer to stay at Marriott hotels. I don't think Marriott has particularly marvelous properties. They're not grand or elegant. They're certainly not chic or trendy. But they are wonderfully consistent from market to market when it comes to certain criteria. In short, they are a real service brand.

In a service industry such as hotels, certain elements define the brand more than others. Among them:

The physical plant. Marriott will never win any awards for attractive architecture. In fact, Marriott's hotels are about the most functional buildings I have ever seen. But that's the point. They work for the business traveler, their primary customer. Marriott has positioned itself neither as a luxury hotel nor as a budget hotel but as a respectable, clean place that understands the needs of its key customer group. The physical plant screams the brand.

Amenities. Marriott did its homework and discovered that the business traveler has rather simple needs. A desk with a phone and a data port for a PC, a health club, and a restaurant that won't poison you (talk about low expectations). The brand creates an expectation that these amenities will be met at each Marriott I stay in. By and large that expectation is met. Brands that fail are those that overpromise and underdeliver. Note throughout this case study how simple Marriott's promises are.

Service. Service is perhaps the one area where a brand can exceed expectations. I'll give an example from a Marriott experience to illustrate my point.

My wife and I were in New York City as part of a combined business and pleasure trip. We had checked out of the hotel and were stuck in traffic in the Lincoln Tunnel when we got into that predictable conversation of "who has the plane tickets." After five minutes of playing the *"you* have them, no *you* have them" game, we of course came to the conclusion that *neither* of us had them. They were in fact somewhere back in the hotel room from which we had just checked out.

Not that I'm a pessimist, mind you, but the possibility that our tickets would be anywhere on the surface of the planet seemed to me to be highly unlikely. But just to amuse myself, I got to a telephone and called the hotel. No surprise when the front desk said, no, they didn't have any tickets, but they would check with housekeeping anyway.

I thought finding the tickets would be enough of a shocker, but how they helped me get them back was the true measure of service—the delivery on their promise. Totally unprompted, the desk clerk asked me over the phone for my destination that evening and my anticipated time of arrival. When I got there, there was a message from the clerk. I returned the call, and she gave me three options for getting the tickets back. I chose to have them messengered to me that night. She implemented the decision and thanked me again for staying at the hotel.

Also note that the person who originally fielded my call was the one who handled the entire matter. I didn't get transferred to the customer relations desk, the general manager, or Bill Marriott for that matter. Their workforce is obviously empowered to deliver on the promise.

Forget what I said about surprises. In service, there are no limits. But if you are going to use service as the basis of your healthcare brand, understand that the standards have been set, not just by Marriott, but by customers who have experienced exceptional surprises. The service satisfaction barrier rises every time a customer has an exceptional experience from anyone, anywhere.

Price. Marriott's pricing reflects its overall position. Not high, not low—but when you get the bill, you say, "That seems pretty fair to me." Marriott appears to have found that elusive "I-got-value" conclusion that so many purchasers seek today.

Location. They have distribution that meets my needs. They're convenient.

Perks. While the elements I have talked about are part of what constitutes a service brand, often you have to do more, still, to consistently acknowledge your best customers. Marriott's not blind to that and has established several programs for its most frequent users. Admittedly, healthcare doesn't want to reward people because they're sick often—obviously, the best reward is good health—but healthcare also has to realize that individuals with chronic conditions *are* going to be repeat users who will be constantly searching for a solution to their medical problems.

The IDN Challenge

It's no easy task to build a brand out of a collection of the acquired properties and disparate users. You have to reinvent cultures, modify physical facilities, and build a central information infrastructure—hardly an overnight project.

To show you how hard it is, I'll relate a personal health story. My mother, age 86 at the time, was in the hospital for some fairly uncomplicated surgery.

She went to a suburban Chicago hospital that had been advertising that the people there were going to pay attention to our needs and respond to them. I was encouraged by that and looked forward to a positive experience for my mother and her "favorite visitor."

While waiting for Mom to return to her room, a chipper young woman strolled by with a cart and offered me a selection of complimentary refreshments. I was so bowled over by the hospitality I almost forgot to make my choice. Hey, I thought, this place is delivering on its promise.

Don't worry, it didn't last long. When my mother failed to appear in her room two hours after they sent her up from recovery, I questioned a nurse at the station about her whereabouts. Unfortunately, I got blasted with a "how should I know?" response, "Can't you see I'm busy?"

The promise of the brand went "poof." I'm not telling this story to be critical of the organization, but rather to illustrate how hard it is to deliver on a branding promise.

Whether you choose to be a Marriott, a Ritz Carlton, or some other brand is not that important. But making the decision—and the commitment—to build and support a true brand is one of the most critical decisions in healthcare leadership today. Can your IDN emulate a Marriott? If it does, you have a service brand.

The market will provide a greater probability of success to those who conquer the branding challenge. It is likely to equally punish those who do not.

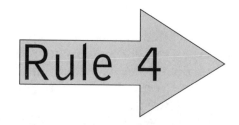

Rule 4

If You're Merging Facilities, Initially Maintain Some of Your Original Brand Identity

How many of the mergers occurring today do you think will last forever? Probably not as many as some would like. In fact, we're already seeing the demise or fracturing of networks throughout the country.

If the merger experiences of other industries are true harbingers for healthcare, then the future isn't very rosy. Securities Data Corporation, Newark, New Jersey, estimates that $659 billion worth of mergers took place in all industries in 1996, up considerably from the $519 billion of the previous year.

Mercer Management Consulting, New York, did a separate study of more than 300 big mergers over the past ten years. Its findings: that in the three years following the deals, 57 percent of the merged firms lagged behind their industries in terms of total returns to shareholders. The rate appears to be higher over the longer term.

What causes mergers to fail? The consensus from several sources seems to be that too much emphasis is placed on the deal itself and not enough attention is paid to "what happens next." Culture, protocol, and technology clashes often flare into internal battles in which the hunter is also the victim.

Admittedly, not all of healthcare is driven by the same dynamics as publicly traded companies. But in many ways hospital acquisition efforts often have been like hostile takeovers forced by economic reality. Early scores by healthcare CEOs on their experiences with mergers suggest that the whole acquisition strategy may be challenged in the not-too-distant future.

According to "U. S. Hospitals and the Future of Healthcare," a study conducted by Deloitte and Touche in 1996, only 7 percent of surveyed healthcare executives reported that they had "reduced or eliminated" services after becoming part of a larger system.

Although some successes have occurred in combining administrative services, the report continued, activity beyond that is limited. Only 8 percent of the healthcare executives said they combined emergency services or inpatient units.

And even more telling, these executives reported a lack of understanding among physicians about the role of managed care and its effect on their organizations.

Not the kind of data to suggest that all relationships are here to stay.

As unfortunate as that may be, it is a fact of business life: some deals just go bad. So what happens to the institution that abandons its current brand equity in favor of jumping on NewCo's bandwagon and then sees the deal go south? It gets to struggle to build awareness and preference all over again. Here's a case in point.

Two modest-sized hospital systems in the Midwest came together for a merger. Any way you looked at the complement of skills and services, the merger made sense. One hospital, which wanted to show its commitment to the venture, agreed to drop all of its institutional promotion and to throw its support behind the effort to create the new brand.

The other hospital chose to support the NewCo brand but also to continue to maintain a presence for itself.

Guess what happened? Conflicts over power and money eventually crumbled the deal, and each institution went back to the market with its original brand. Unfortunately, the hospital that had dropped out of the market during the initial merger activity suffered greatly. Research showed that the brand had lost both awareness and preference. The other system had retained its strength. The system that dropped from the market faced the unpleasant task, not of starting over, but of being in some vague, undefined position. In fact, starting over with a new name might have proved the wiser course.

We can make several arguments for maintaining the local brand: strong community identity and fundraising are just two of them. If NewCo doesn't have a clear message or a cogent strategy, then the case for maintaining local brand identity is irrefutable. Why give up equity for nothing in return?

There is always a huge rush to get NewCo to the market as soon as possible. But often its message is half-baked and the strategy unclear even to the authors. Networks in their early stages are struggling to integrate basic operations, so why burden them with the need to make marketing promises that they surely cannot deliver?

Many systems have found that an evolution to a new super brand has worked and makes good sense. Columbia/HCA is just one example. Its naming strategy has evolved from an identification line, "General Hospital, a Columbia/HCA hospital," to a clear national brand, "Columbia/General Hospital." They dropped the HCA reference from hospital names for a more singular "Columbia" identity.

Note that Columbia did not launch its major branding campaign until several years after it was on the acquisition trail. It seeded the market with the Columbia name for years, but until it was ready to tell people what the brand was all about, it kept its profile pretty low. Once it decided that it wanted to be seen as "a different kind of hospital," it pursued that position aggressively. Court records from its recent trademark challenge from Columbia University, as reported in the September 23, 1996 issue of *Modern Healthcare*, indicate that Columbia is spending more than $100 million annually on advertising, and one can presume that the bulk of that is being used for its branding initiative.

Columbia's initiative is worth reviewing, not so much because it's a brilliant strategy, but because it was executed as a single idea that was consistently delivered in the market. For Columbia, the local brand became less relevant and it fell into a second position for attention. The local brand became the legacy, not the promoted brand (example: Columbia/LaGrange Hospital). It's a smart play even if you don't agree with the message or the company.

It's interesting to see the Columbia brand now being moved to a secondary identifier since the management debacle of 1997. To use the branding models discussed earlier, Columbia has gone from a GE strategy to Nabisco.

Positions Change in Dynamic Markets

Positioning is a dynamic, not static, exercise. Federal Express corporation found that overnight delivery had to be extended first geographically to include global service. Then as competition expanded, the company found that price and service options were the new thresholds for success. "Absolutely, positively overnight" was no longer enough. The market wanted more and Federal Express had to change to meet the demands.

Who better than Columbia/HCA knows about the volatility of positioning in healthcare. Their aggressive move to be known as a "different kind of healthcare company" proved to be their shortfall. Where do they go from here?

That's tough to answer, but they have positioned themselves so far out of the mainstream that they'll need a ton of creative magic to find a credible, useful position. There's reason to believe that the Columbia/HCA name is so badly damaged that it may not be salvageable.

To avoid the peril of losing your identity prematurely, get hold of a clear and cogent strategy that specifies the direction you want for the new entity and plan to move it there. If you are not convinced that the plan can be executed as proposed, consider a parallel promotion preserving your brand.

The market can wait for an IDN's introductory message. If you're not going to say anything worth remembering, why say it?

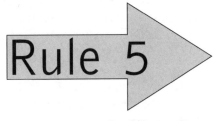

Rule 5

Your New Selling Season Is Called "Open Enrollment"

Seldom has healthcare been considered a seasonal business. But managed care may be changing that. It is creating a season that is to healthcare what Christmas is to retailers—a make-or-break period.

More and more consumers are making a critical choice once a year during "open enrollment"—that annual employee benefits frenzy when workers in large companies choose their health plan for the coming year. If you're not allocating your resources accordingly, you could be missing a big opportunity that won't repeat itself for another year.

Let's look at the numbers.

In 1995, approximately 73 percent of the employed population received its healthcare through managed care, according to "The New Dominance of Managed Care: Insurance Trends in the 1990s," a study that appears in the January/February 1997 issue of *Health Affairs*. A 1997 study by New York–based William M. Mercer Inc. indicated that only 22 percent of surveyed employers are offering just a single type of plan. Essentially that means that once a year, about 78 percent of the employed adults in this country either choose or reconfirm who will provide them with care for the coming 12 months.

Your goal, of course, is to be on the plan they select. And that's why open enrollment is such a critical time. If consumers select a plan in which you participate, you've essentially made the short list. If not, you're out.

The question is, how do you deploy your tactics and resources for this seemingly critical event? A reasonable approach is to create a matrix showing spending levels against penetration levels of managed care (see Table 5.1). The higher the level of managed care, the higher the proportionate spending for open enrollment.

The figures in Table 5.1 are guidelines, mind you, and subject to broad interpretation. Allocate as your market, your organization, and your overall strategy dictate.

Not Just an Advertising Expense

Marketing expenditures for open enrollment do not necessarily translate directly into advertising. Because contracting shifts from year to year, advertising can play a valuable role in informing current users and want-to-be users about the health plans in which you participate. Unfortunately, this form of advertising is more difficult to track than programs that have a direct message-response orientation, but the logic for advertising during this period is pretty compelling if you are in a Stage III or IV market.

Table 5.1 Budget Allocations for Open Enrollment Activities

MCO Development (Penetration)	Percent Open Enrollment Marketing Expenditures
≤10%	0
11–25%	15–20
26–40%	35–40
41% or more	75–80

Other forms of marketing activity are equally important. An essential and usually overlooked group during this period are the physicians and the physicians' offices. As we all know, the most pressing question among consumers during open enrollment is, "Can I keep my physician?" We generally make the consumer do all the work to answer that question and do little to help them stay.

Focus on the Physician Office

The physician setting as a marketing strategy for open enrollment needs to be explored. The activities need not be elaborate—a simple direct mail program from physician to patients encouraging them to "make sure you choose a plan in which I participate"—can be a powerful retention tool.

Similarly, the office staff can be trained to field the avalanche of phone calls about plan participation, office hours, and other benefits during this period. Even a simple tent card in the waiting room can alert patients to a list of participating plans or an invitation to "talk to us about your health plan coverage" can be effective.

Even physicians need to be made more aware of the opportunity that open enrollment provides. Inviting questions or helping patients understand the importance of maintaining continuity of care can help increase or retain members.

The tactics are many. The key is to make the physician and the physician's staff active partners in the enrollment process.

Cutting Through a Confused Market

Business consultant Tom Peters is widely quoted as saying, "Out of chaos comes opportunity." It's advice that would seem to apply to open enrollment as well.

Portability of benefits is increasing, as well as new self-choice products such as medical savings accounts. While the intent of these innovations is to provide more coverage to more individuals, they are more likely to increase confusion among an already confused population. Is it the role of the IDN to be the educator—to guide the market through the swamp? That's a difficult business decision to answer, because there is no guarantee that the individual counseled will become a member. But the opportunity to capture and retain the unaligned patient is growing.

The key is to recognize and seize the potentially huge opportunity of open enrollment. Miss the window and you'll miss the market.

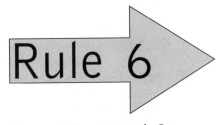

Rule 6

Your Managed Care Contract Is No More Than a Hunting License

The word to remember here is **pull-through**. Conventional wisdom has long held that if you get the contract, you've won the battle. But that's hardly the case. Even within a contract there is no guarantee you'll get any members. You are still competing for members who must choose one of *your* physicians and use *your* services from the other providers offered in the plan.

Thus pull-through—getting the member to select your physicians and hospitals—becomes the operative strategy. If you don't pull the member through to your IDN, the contract has no value. Look at it as a hunting license, and your return should increase.

Many of the chapters/rules in this book address how pull-through can be accomplished (customer service, etc.). But you might consider some of the less obvious ways to influence marketshare.

In the previous chapter, we talked about a pull-through strategy during open enrollment using the physician and the physician office. While that is an effort that certainly needs emphasis, it is also important to look at ongoing marketing behavior.

One area often overlooked for pull-through is the employer worksite.

The Value of the Worksite

Worksite programs for screening and prevention have been in existence for years, and among many they're thought to be no longer effective. But let's revisit and recast them to see if they might not have another life to offer.

The conclusion to an article in the December 1996 *Business and Health,* titled "Can Employers See Beyond Price?" talked about a surprising absence of preventive programs in the workplace despite some overwhelming evidence of their success.

"Nearly nine out of ten respondents have never conducted on site screenings for hypertension or high cholesterol," cited the article, "and fewer than three percent offer them now; more than eight in ten haven't tried smoking cessation or weight loss programs. Only about one in 10 has an in house gym or subsidizes participation in off site programs, despite solid evidence of the benefits of regular exercise." The findings are among larger employers (20–499 employees and 500 or more).

The historical problem, of course, is that no one wants to pay for these types of activities. Employers will admit to their value, but committing money to identify them is clearly another matter—and usually a deal killer.

Worksite programs might benefit from a little imagination. Community Hospitals Indianapolis (CHI), for example, has a refreshing program for employers that shows some creativity and results. CHI has developed three programs for employers that take health promotion beyond the world of cholesterol screenings. Each is customized to the needs of the individual, depending on that individual's interest in improving or maintaining his or her health.

By applying a little creativity to a somewhat burned-out strategy, CHI has found an attractive way to engage employers and their employees. More important, they are showing that they can indeed change behaviors.

One of the programs, called "Picture This," uses an improvisational theater group. Before the performance the actors are given some key words and issues pertaining to the organization's culture. During their improv skit, they present situations pertaining to health and to the organization. At key points, the action stops, and the actors turn to the audience and start asking questions. It's a true interactive session.

Other programs at CHI focus on helping people come to a clearer definition of "health." They consider the environment in which they are working to determine what might be considered a strength or weakness related to health. As Daniel Hodgkins, executive director of Health Promotion at CHI, says, "We look at health as a combination of body, mind, and spirit. Using this framework, we can recognize as 'healthy' even a person who is, for example, a bit overweight and smokes, but is an active positive force in the community."

CHI reports a very positive reaction to the program from local businesses, but the typical reluctance to fund them. The challenge, even to the creative mind, is to demonstrate the short-term benefits of the program.

Clinical Strategies

Not all programs need be held in the public arena. In fact, clinical approaches may prove to hold greater value to the health plan and create a pull-through of a different nature. Here are a few to consider.

Case Management for High-Risk Members

IDNs should be able to make an outstanding argument for their ability to provide case management for high-risk members. The sheer notion of integration creates a compelling platform through which to develop a case management approach.

The key of course is to link the IDN's main clinical areas with the medical needs of the health plan members. That shouldn't be difficult. Start with one or two areas and build a portfolio of programs from there.

HEDIS Compliance Support Programs

HEDIS (Health Plan Employer Data and Information Set) and HEDIS 3.0, plus other forms of accreditation, are fundamental to health plan survival. Without them health plans simply can't compete.

The cost of documenting and implementing many accreditation programs is high, of course, but such efforts create another opportunity for the IDN to create a better partnership with health plans.

HEDIS, for one, requires health plans to demonstrate how they are serving the preventive needs of their members in particular areas. Five of the initial areas include:

- cholesterol screenings;
- diabetic retinal screenings;
- pediatric immunizations;
- mammograms; and
- cervical cancer screenings.

Other areas are reportedly under consideration, and we can expect them to be on the list in the near future.

Those health plans that are IPA (independent practice association) models have a particularly difficult time providing those areas of service because they have so little control over their physician members. Group models, on the other hand, are in a better position to offer the services because they can exert greater control.

An IDN might consider creating a HEDIS compliance package as part of a value-added component to its contracting. HEDIS compliance can be expensive to the plan, but it usually is part of the IDN's stable of existing services. The needs of the health plan can be best served by the IDN—*your* IDN. Sounds like an opportunity.

Disease Management Resource Group

Among the many long-term considerations for managing the healthcare of members is the notion of "disease management." It's a somewhat self-defining term. The goal is to manage the disease and the member closely and rigorously, thus lowering exposure to costly procedures. Disease management uses a range of strategies from education to compliance to reach its desired results.

Historically, disease management was the purview of the pharmaceutical industry. But in offering the programs to health plans, the drug manufacturers found a high degree of skepticism. Plans believed that the manufacturers were creating programs that were more self-serving than beneficial to the plan.

IDNs may have the opportunity to take the higher ground and offer their clinical expertise again as a value-added service. Disease management programs can be customized to the needs of the plan and the integrated skills of the network. At whatever level disease management is eventually offered, it can serve to keep the focus on quality patient care and overall costs. Both the plan and the provider can learn from each other in what may be the beginning of a more lasting partnership.

Miami-based PhyMatrix Corporation has used this strategy so successfully that they have now spun off their disease management activities into a separate company.

The Role of the Brand

Another key element in pull-through is your brand strategy. While we know there is a sizable group of "shoppers" for healthcare, we should keep in mind that an equal number of couch potatoes are simply going to check a box based on the line of least resistance.

Differentiating your network each year before the open enrollment window opens is as important as engaging in the actual pull-through activities. Clearly positioning yourself among consumers before open enrollment is an essential "pre-sell" activity. Don't assume that during open enrollment you will have enough time for effectively getting your positioning message to cut through all the noise in the market and stick in the mind of your hoped-for enrollees. One health plan operating in California reportedly says it has reaped huge success simply because its name begins with the letter *A*, putting it at the head of the list. Consumers are choosing it for little more reason than that.

Open enrollment is a hunting season. Choose your weapons wisely.

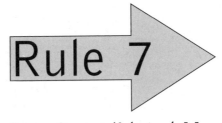

Rule 7

In a Consolidated Market, Re-examine Your Notion of Market Segmentation

It's clear that we are now in a consumer-driven market. Consumers are demanding choice, and employers and their health plans are giving it to them. The tight controls of early managed care activities seem to be fading. Plans such as United HealthCare of Minneapolis, Minnesota, are now merchandizing the fact that members can choose practically any provider they want. Even healthcare futurist Jeff Goldsmith agrees. Writing in the November/December 1996 *Healthcare Forum Journal*, Goldsmith says, "The reality is that employers and consumers are asking for something very different: a seemingly incongruous mixture of broad choice and economic discipline."

While we may think of highly "managed" markets as limiting choice, the preponderance of point-of-service (POS) plans (13 percent of U.S. plans in 1995) is actually expanding it. We are also seeing the Kaisers and the Group Healths turning to POS plans to broaden their reach. Choice will increase and people will exercise it.

A market that offers choice demands a segmentation response.

The industry once thought of itself as a mass marketer, but few industries can survive with just a broad stroke over the market. Segmentation—the ability to deliver a highly focused product and message to a specific audience—must be the strategic mainstay of IDN marketing.

Historically, segmentation has been executed along product lines. Morristown Hospital of Morristown, New Jersey, found that demographic segmentation worked. Rather than take its cardiology services to the mass market, it decided to focus on women over the age of 40. The results supported the decision. In less than two years, Morristown increased its female cardiac business by six percentage points and moved into the "most-preferred" position among women for cardiac services, beating nearby New York City hospitals hands down.

While we have traditionally looked at segmentation along demographic lines, the new market suggests that new segments are out there to identify and understand. There is certainly cross-over and intermingling among the groups, but the key idea here is to rethink your market beyond the traditional "women age 35+ with household incomes over $25,000." Alternate segments include:

Shoppers and non-shoppers. A major national insurance company conducted its own research to see how it could segment the market. Among the several buyer segments it identified, two large groups emerged: the shopper and the non-shopper. The shopper group accounted for about 14 percent of the market—a size not large enough to dominate but at least worth a look.

Some individuals—the shoppers—truly examine all of their options, review the networks, and make an informed decision. They require a great deal of specific information to help them compare the offerings. Shoppers may also be seeking additional services beyond what a plan provides in an uncapitated revenue stream.

The non-shoppers are probably going to make decisions based on familiarity with the brand; the shoppers will seek value. Couch potatoes will buy familiarity.

A shopper/non-shopper segmentation may reveal new products, new money, and new members.

Members and nonmembers. If you are in a highly managed market, you essentially have two consumer groups: the ones for which you have responsibility and the ones for which you don't. And, as we discussed in other parts of this book, each requires a different strategy.

Members must be retained. Nonmembers need to be recruited. Which group is most important? Most attainable?

The well and the chronically ill. Enough databases are available now to help a provider identify the chronically ill members of the community. According to an annual survey by Lincoln, Nebraska-based National Research Corporation, approximately 89.5% of households in America include at least one member with one or more chronic conditions. You can project the health of your community's population based on surveys, or you can even buy mailing lists of individuals who have identified themselves as having any number of problems. If you are still being reimbursed for treating the chronically ill, then a disease-state strategy makes sense.

The so-called "well market" is another market, if an elusive one. As obvious as it seems, the well market is interested in, well, staying healthy. And that's how it needs to be reached: with frequent messages about prevention and the extremely important notion of self-care. Segment your market accordingly.

Adolescents. Adolescents, like seniors, make up an age-specific group that needs attention. Admittedly the teen group is not new to American demography. But it appears that it has been a greatly overlooked and perhaps underserved market.

According to the 1994 National Health Interview Survey (U.S. Department of Health and Human Services), approximately 30.5 million adolescents ages 12–19 live in this country. And they have chronic conditions just like every other segment.

And here's something: many of us probably think that juvenile diabetes is the prevalent disease among teenagers, but it's not. According to the survey, only 97,000 adolescents are afflicted with juvenile diabetes. Other disease states among this population rank considerably higher.

Unfortunately, the literature contains very little that identifies levels of treatment for this group. One study identified what happens to adolescents who don't receive care. In a December 1996 article "Health Status of Well vs. Ill Adolescents" in the *Archives of Pediatric Adolescent Medicine*, Barbara Starfield and colleagues wrote that acutely ill teenagers reported more physical discomfort, minor illnesses, and lower physical fitness than the "normal" group. They also reported more limitations of activity, long-term medical disorders, and dissatisfaction with their health overall.

While their medical needs for today are obvious, one should also consider adolescents as prospects for long-term loyalty. Investing in this segment today could yield high membership numbers down the road.

The boomers. Once known for their youthfulness and high energy levels, the baby boom generation (those born between

Table 7.1   Prevalence of Disease Among Adolescents in the United States

Migraine headaches	1,127,000 individuals
Kidney trouble	238,000
Heart disease	1,265,000
Hypertension	189,000
Hay fever, allergies	4,837,000

Source: *Vital and Health Statistics*, 1994. U.S. Department of Health and Human Services, Series 10: Data from the National Health Interview Survey, No. 193.

1946 and 1965) are finding fallibility with every new ache and pain. They are realizing that their seemingly perpetual fountain of youth is sputtering dry. And along with the sputter comes the inevitable array of things that don't work as well as they used to.

And important to note here is that the boomer generation will grow a staggering 71 percent by the year 2010, one of the largest-growing segments of the U.S. population.

But the boomers appear different from those aging populations that preceded them. To the boomer generation, the problems of aging are seen more as nuisances, issues that can be handled rather than something that becomes "chronic." This view represents a growing opportunity for providers. More important, boomers appear to have the resolve, the education, and the all-important financial resources to be aggressive on their own behalf. In short, they represent an ideal target market for healthcare organizations.

Appealing to this group will take a more sophisticated approach to product-line development than providers have followed in the past. Boomers feel more empowered, seek greater participation, and are aware of a wide range of treatment options both traditional and otherwise. Find their proverbial hot button, and the rewards should be plentiful.

Other segments can and must exist. The marketer's challenge is to look at the world in a nontraditional way for a nontraditional solution. The rewards are there to reap.

Rule 8

Nothing Is More "Relationshippy" Than Healthcare: Maximize It

Healthcare is the epitome of one-on-one marketing. But most approach it solely as a mass marketing event. Unless the two strategies reconcile themselves, marketing will become futile. And gigantically wasteful.

One-on-One Marketing: The Rewards

The rewards for the one-on-one marketer can be significant. According to a study by Boston-based Bain & Company, a typical *Fortune* 500 company has annual growth of 2.5 percent. By retaining an additional 5 percent of its customers, growth will triple to 7.5 percent and profits increase by 25 percent. In addition, says the report, increasing customer retention by just 2 percent can decrease costs by as much as 10 percent. Relationship marketing—the process whereby you maximize the potential of each individual customer—can be a key in attaining those financial goals.

Relationship marketing has proved outstandingly successful in other industries along with healthcare. According to a 1996 report on database marketing (*The Cowles Report*, October 1996), consumer product companies have made significant investments—and have seen equal returns—in database marketing. The ranking of U.S. companies by size of investment in database marketing:

1. Kraft Foods;
2. Ralston Purina;
3. Phillip Morris;
4. SmithKline Beecham;
5. Kimberly-Clark;
6. Nestlé;
7. Bristol Myers Squibb; and
8. RJ Reynolds, Sandoz Consumer, and Sara Lee (three-way tie).

It shouldn't surprise you too much that three of the top eight companies are in the healthcare industry. Indeed, the *Cowles Report* points out that database activity among drug companies has increased 400 percent since FY 1992–1993, including a 54 percent jump in FY 1996 alone. Clearly, healthcare is seizing database marketing as a key initiative. The category's increase in database marketing activity is nearly twice that of the combined total of database marketing activity for all packaged goods companies tracked.

Perhaps healthcare has learned the lessons of other groups that have used relationship marketing strategies. Marriott Hotels, considered by many to have the best relationship marketing program in the industry, has found that its Honored Guests members spend two-and-a-half times more at Marriott locations than they did as customers before joining the program.

Just what is relationship marketing for healthcare? In its simplest form it is being proactive in much the same way that dentists, veterinarians, and retailers are when they send us reminders that we need to have our teeth cleaned, our dogs groomed, or the oil in our cars changed. While it appears on the surface that these companies are out to get more business, they are building on an earlier encounter, sustaining the relationship through a program that provides valuable information, and creating an economic exchange. These businesses understand that a customer has a lifetime value with significant return on investment.

The Difference Between Relationship Marketing and Database Marketing

There's an important difference in approach between relationship marketing and database marketing.

Relationship marketing is almost a self-defining term. It works to *understand* and, most important, to *anticipate* the needs of the customer. Relationship marketing is characterized by a combination of service and promotional strategies.

Database marketing is a little less personal and subscribes to the theory that people with similar tastes and lifestyles will behave in a similar manner. It *works by the numbers* by listing a set of buyer attributes and then seeking individuals who have those same attributes. Banks are very good at database marketing. They create a profile of, say, purchasers of vacation homes and then lay that profile over their checking account customers. When there is a match, the person holding that checking account receives promotional material on vacation home loans.

A Lesson from Car Maker Saturn

Saturn understands the lifetime value of a customer. A typical dealership earns more than half of its revenues from its parts and service business, but 95 percent of the typical automotive advertising budget is directed at new car sales. The remaining 5 percent—what we'll call loyalty dollars—has an incredible financial return over the life of the customer and the business. Saturn spends that 5 percent on programs that target existing owners for preventive and maintenance programs, and these owners generate half the Saturn dealer's revenues.

IDNs, because of their size and complexity, are ideal companies for relationship marketing programs. First, they have huge databases of hundreds of thousands of users. A profile can be created from these databases and various segments established. But because an IDN has diverse properties, it can market around each entity or it can cross-sell from one facility or service to another in the IDN community. It can be much easier to drive a wellness center from an IDN database of several hundred thousand familiar users than to try to mine an untested, disloyal population.

The working of relationship marketing is subject to the needs and resources of the sponsor. Many marketing executives in the service industry are taking a new and refreshing view of what constitutes relationship marketing. The popular "frequent user" concept is falling out of favor for some (just look at the airlines!) primarily because of high maintenance costs and a concern that rising consumer expectations will force purveyors of this strategy to spend even more on incentives in the future.

One Customer at a Time

A different tack, and perhaps one applicable to the healthcare industry, is to focus on maximizing customer satisfaction at the time of the encounter. In other words, focus on making each encounter exceed a customer's expectations. It's a clear tie to a service strategy, and it appears to work.

Ritz-Carlton Hotels offer one approach. They maintain an extensive database of their customers, noting preferences for just about everything. An electric iron in the room, the use of turndown service, even car preference for a ride to the airport is noted in the customer's record. Employees carry customer preference pads with them, noting needs of customers that are later entered into their record.

It's unlikely that providers will ever match that level of service. That's not the point. What is important is that frequent customers have needs and wants that influence their satisfaction and ultimately their return business. While a provider is not going to have an iron in the room, it can apply this approach by noting some of the important needs of its high-use patients. Does the patient need transportation? How about assistance in getting from reception to the treatment area? Special considerations at home? All of these concerns are appropriate for a provider to address.

With IDNs investing millions of dollars in new management information systems, including the networks' marketing needs in its design and function will provide considerable value.

Ritz-Carlton delivers its relationship marketing program primarily at the time of check-in—recognizing customers' individual needs and rewarding them with room upgrades and the like. The hotel immediately communicates to customers that they are important and proves it with some type of reward. It should come then as no surprise that of the Ritz-Carlton's 500,000 annual customers recorded, 60 percent are repeating their visits.

Applications Beyond the Consumer Market

The consumer/patient, as we all know, is hardly your only "customer." Building and maintaining satisfactory relations—loyalty programs—can be applied to any customer group. Physicians, managed care organizations and employer subscribers are as likely to be candidates as the consumer. Budget Rental Car Corporation focused its relationship marketing on travel agents nationwide. Through a system of recognition and rewards known as Book Smart, Budget was able to enroll 25,000 travel agents in its program. Travel agents account for 70 percent of Budget's business. A recent analysis showed that Book Smart agents have five times greater revenues than nonparticipating agents. Perhaps there is a similar application among insurance brokers and other referral sources.

Healthcare Applications

In healthcare, a notion—long floated but rarely exercised—acknowledges that as your body ages its medical needs change. And that along the way providers have an opportunity to build and sustain a relationship by educating the individual on what to expect as each stage of the life cycle approaches and then guiding the person through that stage and into the next through appropriate interventions, education, and therapies. I developed this strategy in the mid '80s as part of some work for Baxter International. It was called "Lifecycle Management," and it appears to be an idea whose time has arrived.

Earlier I discussed the generation of baby boomers as an emerging segment worth pursuing. If you're in your '40s or beyond, you, too, may have noticed that some of your parts are not functioning quite as they used to. Most likely you are also starting to look over the horizon of your next decade and are beginning to realize that, not too far from now, even fewer things will work as well as they once did.

Would you see value in having someone guide you through those changes? Not just at the time that a treatment is called for, but in a more fundamental, less clinical, proactive way? Research, not to mention common sense, says that men and women across a range of income groups and ages would appreciate such guidance.

Relationship marketing is not necessarily an expensive, or for that matter inexpensive, strategy to execute. It can cost a sizable amount to create a database and maintain it, but as healthcare benefits become more and more portable, the value of sustaining a relationship increases dramatically. Your marketing dollar has a higher yield. It takes far fewer dollars to maintain a customer than to acquire a new one.

The Cost Side

Healthcare applications of relationship and database marketing are both in their infancy. Most of the database examples come from health plans looking to increase their share of the Medicare risk market.

DiMark Marketing of Langehorn, Pennsylvania, considered by many to be a leader in database marketing, has helped unravel some of the cost issues related to database marketing. According to DiMark's experience, the cost of acquiring a Medicare risk member can range from as little as $200 to over $1,000. The range of per-member costs demonstrates that a wide range of tactics are used to acquire a member, and that those tactics spring from a database strategy that targets a very diverse audience.

Database and relationship marketing do not imply cost savings. But they do promote efficiencies and they provide a clearer means of tracking results than do traditional broad-based programs. The one thing these programs do not do is build brands. They help *harvest* the demand for a brand via a specific product offering. It's a classic case of needing both marketing strategies to succeed. One enhances the other; it does not supplant it.

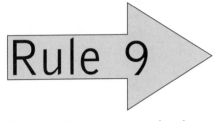

Rule 9

Get a New Vocabulary

"Soccer mom" was voted Word of the Year by the American Dialect Society beating out "alpha geek" for the number one slot.

—As reported in *USA Today,* January 6, 1997

I've been in the healthcare business for over 20 years, and I still pause for a moment every time I hear the terms "morbidity" and "mortality." I know that one of them is worse than the other, but I really have to think about it before I understand that mortality is the end game and morbidity is an index of problems.

But our industry talks to people freely and without explanation about our "mortality and morbidity" rates, our "ALOS," and our "continuum of care." Do we seriously think people understand what we're talking about? It's no wonder people find healthcare such a scary, often incomprehensible experience.

The New English Language

Like it or not, our fast-paced society has evolved its own form of communication, often departing drastically from the

English language and its basic syntax. The American Dialect Society resoundingly confirmed that fact with "soccer mom" and the hundreds of other neologisms invented every year. Add to that the fact that most goods and services are sold in the media with simple messages that last no more than 30 seconds, and it's clear that to have a discernible, much less a compelling, message, you need to use words that say what they mean to audiences without the time to translate healthcare mumbo jumbo.

The Literacy Issue

In Timothy R. Covington's article "Physical Assessment: The Pharmacist and the Self-Medicating Patient," in the August 1996 *Drug Newsletter*, he cites that approximately 20 percent of the U.S. population are functionally illiterate, and almost 40 percent of some population subsets the same. Because of this, providers have a significant communications challenge. Reading levels are estimated to be between the sixth and tenth grades for 35 percent of the population—and hearing/listening/"grasping" levels are geared to 30-second sound bites.

Trust me. More often than not, you're talking to yourself. You need a new vocabulary.

Business and Health in its March 1997 issue looks realistically at the size of the communication barrier the healthcare industry has created for itself. Citing a survey by Siegal & Gale and Roper Starch Worldwide, the researchers report on levels of comprehension of "health speak" (see table 9.1).

Use of plain English in simple sentences will work quite handily. And although most advisers suggest that you write to a sixth-grade level, you might want to consider setting your sights a little lower, say at fourth-grade levels, to accommodate the wide range of issues, their inherent complexity, and the industry's need to be able to speak to all members of society. States are mandating managed care

Table 9.1 Consumers' Understanding of Healthcare Terms

Term	Consumers Sure of Meaning/ Have a Fairly good idea (%)
HMO	67
Wellness program	54
PPO*	37
Indemnity plan	24
POS	15

Source: Business and Health, March 1997.
*preferred provider organization

Table 9.2 Replaceable Healthcare Phrases

Phrase	Suggested Replacement
Morbidity and mortality	How about "sick" and "died"?
Outcomes data	Talk about impersonal; yikes! Try "Our experience with these situations . . ."
Paradigm	A 1980s buzzword; don't even try to replace it.
Continuum of care	Nobody understands it; nobody has it. Talk about the fact that your physician has more resources to help you.
Healthcare system	"System" repeatedly scores in focus groups as a negative. "Alliance" and "partnership" score well.
Gatekeeper	What gate? Not a self-defining term. Stick to "your personal physician."
Access	Do you mean to insurance, physicians, and/or transportation? Don't even try to explain this one.
Patient-focused care	Where else would care be focused? A good turn of phrase might be "keeping the focus on patient care."

options to the least-educated segment of the population. Sorting out the options is hard enough for the educated population. Imagine the barriers for those less fortunate.

Replace These Phrases

The best place to start your quest for clarity is to dump many of the words you're using now. They're confusing, without benefit, and a hindrance to your ability to connect with the marketplace.

The list of confusing healthcare terms, unfortunately, is endless. Speak clearly and simply. The rewards will be many.

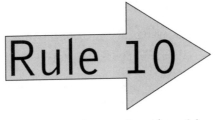

Rule 10

Be Cautious in the Use of Outcomes Data

76 percent of liberals and 87 percent of conservatives believe in miracles

—from a study published in George, *December 1997.*

Conventional wisdom holds that the hospital that scores best on procedures will win the game, that somehow we are a nation that scrutinizes each of our healthcare purchases based on "just the facts, ma'am."

There's a fair amount of evidence to suggest that we buy things by the numbers. We have labeled all our food so we know what we're eating. We rate our mutual funds on their performance. And we can pull up reports on the fuel economy, average maintenance costs, and manufacturer recall records on anything that rides the roads.

It would seem pretty obvious from this behavior that we just need to provide consumers with black-and-white evidence of hospital and physician performance, and once again the decisions will fall in line quite nicely.

However, this conventional wisdom may not be the case, at least not yet.

What Drives Choice?

A study by the Kaiser Family Foundation and the Agency for Health Care Policy and Research (conducted by Princeton Survey Research Associates, October 1996) demonstrated that, in fact, we are far from a nation of rampant consumerism in healthcare.

The study, titled *Americans as Health Care Consumers: The Role of Quality Information,* talked with 2,006 adults about how they choose health plans, physicians, and hospitals.

Not surprisingly, consumers pegged "quality" as their number one selection factor for all three provider groups studied. The studies established early on that consumers do in fact differentiate within each group. Respondents said they saw a "big difference" as follows:

Table 10.1   Consumer Perceptions of Points of Difference Among Providers

Provider	Degree of Difference (%)
Local hospitals	38
Family doctors	37
Health plans	47
MD specialists	28

Clearly, people do see a difference. The logical question becomes: Is the outpouring of clinical data driving these perceptions?

The researchers say "no." According to their data, only about 30 percent of the population uses this type of data to decide on the choice of either a hospital, health plan, or physician. (Interestingly, the study correlated use of performance data in the purchase of new cars and found the percentages to be about the same.) But over 80 percent said they would find such information to be useful if it were made available to them.

Most surprising in the study was the consumers' perception of the most "believable" source of healthcare data. As you might suspect, it's not the healthcare industry.

Cited as "most believable" by respondents was "family and friends." Statistically, the people closest to us in private life are leaders in the "who's best for your health" credibility war. They beat out employers (19 percent "very believable"), physician groups (29 percent), past patients (34 percent), and most certainly the media (5 percent).

From the data provided in the survey, all of the emphasis placed on making it to such honor roles as *U. S. News and World Report's* Top 100 Hospitals seems somewhat misplaced and the distinction rather dubious. Only 11 percent of those surveyed said it would be a major influence in their choice of hospitals.

Other industries have also looked at their notion of outcomes data and have taken a cautious approach. A good example is the airlines.

The Airline Analogy

Note the care with which the airline industry selects the performance data that it uses. Benchmarks such as "on-time arrival," "lost baggage," and complaints per thousand miles flown are readily available. But nowhere do you see their safety records—their mortality and morbidity data—trumpeted in the market. Why? Because it just takes one slight human or mechanical error to wipe out a perfect record. I can't imagine a major airline running an ad saying, "We have the fewest crashes of any major airline." Why should healthcare providers take the same type of risk?

Note how Volvo has positioned itself as the "safe" car without going into any statistical support about the percentage of owners who survive a crash. It shows how people have survived, but it never goes so far as to suggest what the odds of survival would be. Michelin Tires, with its highly memorable baby-in-a-tire ads, has clearly locked up the safety position in its category. But how many of its tires have performed to a given standard? We'll never know.

Is a New "Gold Standard" on the Horizon?

Part of the problem with using data is the cacophony of rating systems and reports. While the National Council of Quality Assessment and the Joint Commission on Accreditation of Healthcare Organizations have clear quality positions among providers, they have little cachet among consumers. But it looks like a gold standard is about to emerge.

If one thinks about the standard-setter for quality rankings in the overall consumer market, it's probably J. D. Power and Associates, Agora Hills, California, as a true "voice of the consumer." The work of this group in the automobile industry is landmark, and its findings carry considerable clout with the consumer. Who hasn't seen how the automotive leaders have leveraged their Power's rating as part of their overall positioning effort?

In 1997, J. D. Power and Associates announced a venture with The Medstat Group, Ann Arbor, Michigan, and the New England Medical Center in Boston, two national healthcare leaders, to bring that same "voice" to the healthcare market by rating health plans in markets throughout the United States. The Power's entrance to the market was clearly a response to "the noise," according to Michael Vollmer, manager of healthcare research at J. D. Power. "There is a need for one clear voice," he said; "That is what we hope to become."

The entrance of J. D. Power and others into to the market is significant for several reasons.

First is the product itself. According to J. D. Power, the product will assess satisfaction among consumers, physicians, and purchasers of healthcare. The group will also gather information on claims, medical records, and encounter data. In addition, the final report also will provide disease-specific information. Citing diabetes as an example, Power reports that its research will show the number of cases each plan has and compare each plan's success in taking care of those patients.

Second, it again demonstrates the power of the brand, which in this case is J. D. Power and Associates. They are well positioned as a premier company in the field. The halo of that reputation will easily carry over to healthcare, a vast wasteland of national sources for quality information.

Put the Data to Use in the Right Arena

There is no escaping the need for outcomes data. Those who purchase healthcare wholesale will demand such information even if they're not quite sure what to do with it. And a measurable portion of the consumer market will demand it as well. But there may be greater wisdom in making the data available rather than promoting them. You never know when "pilot error" will strike.

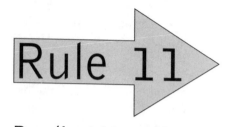

Rule 11

Readjust Your Notion of
Service—the Big and
Perhaps Only True
Opportunity to Differentiate

It shouldn't come as a surprise that Americans see a decline in service across the board. University of Michigan Business School professor Claes Fornell, among others, has documented it.

In 1994 Fornell began the American Consumer Service Index (ACSI), which regularly interviews 16,000 customers of 200 companies in 33 industries. He reported in June 23, 1997 issue of *Newsweek* that indeed our experiences are deteriorating. Using a scale of 1 to 100, he documented the steady decline from 1994.

	1994	1997
Local phone	74.5	70.7
Airlines	79	75
Hospitals	72	67

The only solace here is that consumers' experiences overall are continuing to disappoint.

In any selling proposition, the argument always comes down to one basic question: "So," asks the buyer, "just what makes you different?" As earlier chapters have indicated, that question is becoming particularly difficult for healthcare providers to answer.

Admittedly, hospitals have gone and continue to go to great lengths to talk about their performance, credentials, and network. But rarely is that a slam-dunk strategy. Why? Because while purchasers continually seek a more sophisticated approach to buying, more often than not they come back to one simple criterion: *Were my employees satisfied with the experience?* The provider that can't answer "yes" is out of luck; the one who can expound on and extol the subject is the unanimous winner.

A study among managed care executives, conducted by Foster and Higgins, ranked the managed care organization's (MCO) perceptions of criteria for success. Price, of course, was number one, but racing strongly behind it was member satisfaction at 55 percent.

The important message here is that MCOs really don't have that much contact with their members. The managed care experience is often defined by the member as the relationship and experience he or she has with providers. It's a classic "trickle-up" phenomenon. It looks like this:

Figure 11.1   The Trickle-Up Model of Managed Care

The CEO tells the MCO that
everyone is happy and the MCO gets to
keep the business.

↑

The boss tells the CEO.

↑

They tell their boss.

↑

Members have a positive experience.

This is a greatly simplified model, to be sure, but not without some validity.

For years hospitals have taught the "smile school" approach as a subset of service. The general belief was that if we were nice to people and helped them navigate a hostile environment, they would be more satisfied customers. And by and large they were right. Hospitals that pursued smile strategies saw their patient-satisfaction scores rise. But, inevitably as they did so, another phenomenon occurred. Patient expectations grew.

Expanded Expectations

Several independent studies have confirmed that consumers and patients have redefined what they now consider to be "good service" from a healthcare provider. The good news is that the efforts to be more courteous by the medical and office staff are noticed and appreciated. And by and large the hotel amenities are equally acknowledged.

But according to extensive studies by the Picker Institute, Boston and Press, Ganey Associates of South Bend, Indiana, smile school by itself is no longer enough for patients. Expectations have changed, and providers need to change with them.

In the Picker study about one-third of all hospital and outpatient surgery patients surveyed reported problems getting answers to important questions. In addition, they felt they were not fully informed about the side-effects of medication, warning signs, or the resumption of normal activity. The report went on to say that approximately 28 percent of patients in physician offices felt the same way. Only 4 to 7 percent of patients gave providers low scores for courtesy.

The report concluded that approximately one in every three hospital patients reported having not enough say in their treatment.

Press, Ganey, using its vast database of patient satisfaction reports from 545 hospitals in 44 states, supported the Picker study. Its top four issues were cheerfulness of the hospital, staff concern for privacy, attention paid to special or personal needs, and the degrees to which nurses took health problems seriously. Once again, amenities issues such as food, noise levels, and so forth placed dead last in importance.

A somewhat similar study by the American Hospital Association concluded that America's hospitals are "losing the trust" of their patients, according to a statement by Dick Davidson, AHA president.

This chapter does not suggest that providers are abandoning serious initiatives in order to emphasize courteous service to patients. It does, however, speak to rising expectations of the consumer that must be constantly monitored and resolved. Communication appears to be the new standard of service as defined by the customer.

By now I hope you are starting to link some of the ideas of several of these chapters: the notion of a brand, its singular focus, and the role of satisfaction. If they are all starting to blend together, that's great. None of these elements is independent of the others. They all work in the aggregate to define and differentiate you in the market based on the performance of your enterprise with each customer.

As healthcare benefits become more and more portable, the notion of exclusivity fades and choice becomes the norm. Evidence throughout this book indicates that quality, at least by today's standards, is determined by the customer's experience. And the essence of that experience is communication.

The key is to listen to the market's definition of service and not your own.

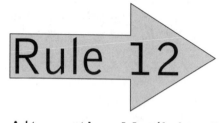

Rule 12

Alternative Medicine Is No Longer a Marketing "Alternative"

Healthcare providers and payors have for years been trying to understand what role, if any, alternative (homeopathic) medicine has in the treatment process. "Is it appropriate? Does it work? Who wants it?" have been among their endless questions.

Today, it looks like their questions are being answered.

Alternative medicine—therapies and procedures that fall outside the traditional definition of allopathic medicine—is not merely arriving, it is bursting into our culture. Integrating such care is no longer a question of "if," but one of "when." And a report in the *New England Journal of Medicine* (January 28, 1993) confirms it. According to author David Eisenberg, an assistant professor of medicine at Harvard Medical School, one-third of surveyed adults had turned to alternative care, mostly for chronic conditions.

The National Institutes of Health (NIH) has divided alternative medicine into seven categories:

1. *Mind-body interventions*
   - Examples: biofeedback, meditation, relaxation techniques

2. *Alternative systems of medical practice*
   - Examples: acupuncture, natural products
3. *Manual healing methods*
   - Examples: acupressure, aromatherapy, chiropractic medicine
4. *Pharmacological and biological treatments*
   - Examples: antioxidants, metabolic therapy
5. *Bioelectromagnetic techniques*
   - Examples: blue light treatment
6. *Herbal medicine*
   - Examples: echinacea, ginger rhizome
7. *Diet, nutrition, and lifestyle*
   - Examples: changes in lifestyle, diet

The numbers are compelling. NIH reports that only between 10 and 30 percent of the world's human healthcare is delivered by conventional, biomedically-oriented practitioners. The remaining 70 to 90 percent relies on self-care and folk principles. Admittedly most of that is outside the United States, but the data do provide a gateway to the size and potential of the acceptance of the discipline.

Other facts at home support the case as well. According to New York City–based Packaged Facts in May 1996's "The Homeopathic Products Market," retail sales of homeopathic remedies reached $230 million in 1995. The market is expected to double by the turn of the century.

As important to any growth-oriented company, the demographics of these alternative medicine consumers are very attractive. The study by Packaged Facts shows users of alternative medicine to be well educated and affluent.

In Search of an Acceptable Form

Alternative medicine is something of a black hole to many individuals both inside and outside of healthcare. The very term "alternative medicine" is conveniently being replaced with "complementary medicine" as the preference of many professionals.

As in any emerging category, the fringe tends to characterize the middle, so herbal teas and unusual therapies find themselves in the same discussion as more acceptable procedures such as acupuncture and chiropractic. But despite the confusion and the clamor, alternative medicine is about to move dead center into the limelight and the revenue stream.

Thanks to the efforts of credible leaders such as Dr. Dean Ornish of Mutual of Omaha, in Nebraska, and Dr. Herbert Benson of the Mind/Body Institute in Boston, efforts to increase the acceptance and use of complementary procedures are gaining significant clinical credibility.

Benson, via his own reports, cites interesting results. Using a population of 7,500 patients at Deaconess Hospital in Boston, the use of relaxation response techniques alone is attributed to producing a 36 percent increase in fertility rate for couples trying to conceive within six months of completing the program. That compares with 17 percent effectiveness for "traditional" treatments.

Benson goes on to predict that providers can reduce overall HMO visits by 50 percent and reduce visits for chronic pain by 30 percent. A projection, indeed, but even if he is half right the savings under capitation are worth considering.

Government and Marketplace Validation

The federal government through the NIH developed the Office of Alternative Medicine in 1994. In 1996, the office awarded $7 million in grants to determine the scientific validity of alternative techniques. Hundreds of studies are coming forth showing definite clinical correlations between mind and body as well as the effectiveness of alternative procedures, for example, in treating pain and hypertension.

And thanks to an increasing demand from consumers, alternative medicine is being accepted by a wider group of payors.

Recent research in "Health Maintenance Organizations and Medicine: A Closer Look" from Landmark Healthcare, Sacramento, California, on the attitudes of managed care members toward alternative medicine yielded even more support for the conventional acceptance of unconventional means. The study showed that 70 percent of managed care executives reported an increase in requests for alternative measures from their members, and 40 percent believed that they would increase enrollment by offering alternative medicine. When queried about their interests in alternative therapies, managed care members gave the ratings shown in Table 12.1.

Early Steps at Integration

Some MCOs already are integrating alternative medicine. Oxford Health Plans of Norwalk, Connecticut, now has a

Table 12.1 Managed Care Members' Interest in Alternative Therapies

Alternative Therapy	Members Interested (%)
Acupuncture	58
Chiropractic	50
Massage therapy	26
Acupressure	21
Biofeedback	21

Source: Landmark Healthcare, Sacramento, CA, 1996.

network of 2,000 credentialed providers of alternative medicine. Other plans such as Kaiser Permanente of Northern California are adding their own benefits programs to include complementary procedures. The State of Washington requires that insurers pay for visits to all categories of healthcare providers licensed by the state. That covers approximately 30 types of caregivers.

Most of the health-plan programs appear to be discounting mechanisms, but nonetheless their very admission into the plans validates them.

Link to the IDN

For the IDN, alternative medicine represents an opportunity to add another dimension to its provider network. At this stage, it may even prove to be a clear point of difference. Because alternative medicine does not appear to be a capitated service, it could also represent a new, unfettered revenue stream.

The wise move would be to find ways to integrate appropriate procedures into existing treatment protocols. Relaxation therapy to improve the childbirth experience and acupuncture to reduce pain in chronic conditions are two areas where use of complementary medicine can either demonstrate improved results or improve patient satisfaction with a therapy.

The more esoteric procedures may need a little more time in the laboratory. Nonetheless, there is sufficient research to validate a trial program and enough economic incentive to build one.

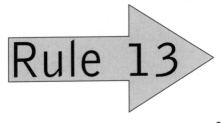

Rule 13

Follow the Consumer for Internet Opportunities

"It's [the Internet] like getting your medical information seated at a bay between a Nobel prizewinner and a pitchman. Let the surfer beware."

—*from the "Health Journal" in the* Wall Street Journal, *December 23, 1996.*

Strategic planners always advise their clients to "skate to where the hockey puck is going." One assumes the hockey puck is "the future." For healthcare marketers, that future could be the Internet.

Few industries in America are as well suited for Internet applications as healthcare. The trouble is, the industry hasn't quite figured out what those applications are.

In fact, many leading companies in America have reassessed their Internet strategies. Today, the thought leaders are saying that the best strategy is to "follow the consumer," meaning that the thoughtful IDN should hold off on major investments until the consumer gives a clearer indication of how he or she wants to use IDN Web site information.

According to *Deja News* as reported in *Yahoo! Internet Life* (February 1997) nearly one-half million hits to medically related news groups occurred in 1996. By 1999, reports *Newsweek*, 34.6 million households in the United States and Canada are expected to be online with a total of 56.7 million households worldwide. The number of hits to healthcare Web sites should increase at a much higher, disproportionate rate.

Meet the "HealthMed Retriever"

A recent study on people's use of the Internet for healthcare provided a somewhat surprising profile of those who use it now and the uses they would like to put it to in the future.

Find/SVP Emerging Technologies Research Group in New York published a study on Internet usage for health and medical information. Here's what they found.

Dubbed "HealthMed Retrievers," the medical/health information group represents approximately 36.7 percent of the general Internet user population (GIUP). The group is expected to grow dramatically as "an additional 43.4 percent of the GIUP plan to begin accessing the Internet's vast health and medical resources within a year."

Of most interest was the *type* of information sought. While it would be easy to say HealthMed Retrievers "want it all" (see Table 13.1), the bigger message is that they see the Internet primarily as a two-way communication vehicle between themselves and their physician.

But the usage of the Internet may be a little less surprising once you look at the demography of the users. According to Find/SVP's report, HealthMed Retrievers are:

- women;
- older, with higher incomes, advanced educations;
- parents with children at home under the age of 18;
- visiting the Web daily and more likely to take in-depth views of the sites they reach;

Table 13.1 Profile of Healthcare Users on the Internet

Areas Visited	Percent That Cited Area as Most Important
Information from MD's office	57
Fitness and stress	55
Diseases	55
Injuries	51
Prescription drugs	49
Diet and food supplements	46
Support groups	46
Health insurance	40
Child development	39

Source: Find/SVP, New York, 1995.

- more likely than the general Internet population to conduct online searches for product information prior to a purchase; and
- likely to have reduced their time spent using print and electronic media.

These same demographics characterize the segment that is the heaviest "shopper" for healthcare services in general. It appears that they are changing media to get their information.

Hundreds of books and articles are out there on how best to use the Internet for healthcare. This chapter/rule isn't about how to construct a Web site; it's about the strategic importance of the Internet.

An Internet Perspective

If we look at how healthcare information fits into the "knowledge thirst" of America, maybe we can come up with a scenario for how it fits into IDN marketing.

Ask any news editor about what their research says is the most sought after topics by consumers, and you'll likely hear "healthcare." But, as we know, healthcare information tends to be rather complex. There are no simple answers to the questions. There's always that "it depends" clause that creeps into any basic inquiry.

Frankly, the Internet is one of the best "it depends" responders available today. Why? Because it allows the reader to drill down a topic and link to other sources of information. In many ways the Internet is becoming the "electronic brochure" of marketing communications. Think about it. Rather than asking people to call you for a free brochure, ask them to visit your Web site with specific information about the topic at hand.

That scenario of course begs that the Web page be more than an electronic billboard. It, like other information sources, must be specific to the needs of the audience.

Let's illustrate how the Internet fits into the overall marketing strategy as opposed to being this tactical thing that hangs out on its own.

Branding
A more global message that differentiates the organization from its competitors. Usually this is a mass media effort using broadcast and other mass media. Messages are brief. Web page supports branding message with additional general information.

Product-Line Advertising
Specific problem/solution messaging. Usually speaks to one's capabilities and expertise. Old way of ending ad: Call for our free brochure. New: Get more information about this procedure on our Web site, register for classes, etc.

Web Site
If integrated into product-line advertising, the Web works to enhance the information discussed in the product-line message. More importantly, it can link the reader to other

healthcare resources within the system or through external sources. The Web site can link readers to physician referral services, class registration, and more.

The more you do to integrate the Web as part of a messaging and capture strategy, the harder it can work for you. If you buy the problem/solution idea fostered elsewhere in this book, this notion should make sense.

Today, the Internet is a marketing mystery. There is a fundamental belief that it has the potential to play an unprecedented role in all aspects of marketing. But finding the true path is expensive and time consuming, and money and time are two resources of measurable scarcity to IDNs. The Internet cannot be ignored, but the wiser course follows the lead of the proven investments of other pioneers.

Rule 14

Work with the Retail Pharmacist . . . Watch Out for the Retail Pharmacist

Can chapters have multiple-choice names? In this case, they can. The role of the retail pharmacist is clearly changing and it needs new definition. Depending on how IDNs and pharmacists act, the chapter title changes. Here's how.

If one were to take a somewhat cynical look at the hierarchy of the delivery of healthcare, we would see the physician at the top, of course, followed by the nurse, and ending with the retail pharmacist. While physicians and nurses have received most of the attention from providers, retail pharmacists have been working quietly to become a more significant player in the delivery of care. And it appears that they are succeeding.

Given their current direction and motivation, the retail pharmacist may prove to be an ideal ally for the IDN—or a menacing competitor.

The New Realities of the Retail Pharmacy

Retail pharmacists represent an important new marketing venue for three simple reasons: the growth of the self-care market, legislative initiatives, and economic necessity. All have the potential for a powerful effect on the delivery of healthcare, and if the trend in managed care continues to move the patient to the most cost-efficient site of care, the retail setting becomes strategically important. The retail pharmacy opportunity is big, it's unexplored, and it's still open to development.

It is also an extremely broad distribution system. Larger U.S. markets can easily have more than 500 retail locations able to supplement, stand in for, or even replace some of the more traditional provider venues. Chicago-based Walgreen Company, a major U.S. chain, has as many as 275 stores in its hometown. That's a considerable network that's either on your side or against you.

The basic behavior of Americans shows how critical the role of the pharmacist is today. According to Timothy R. Covington, PharmD, MS, at Samford University School of Pharmacy, in "Physical Assessment, the Pharmacist and the Self-Medicating Patient," in August 1996 *Drug Newsletter*, there is little doubt that the pharmacist in the managed care environment will be a major player.

Published reports indicate that the average American has one potentially self-treatable problem every three to four days. Approximately 90 percent of the U.S. population considers itself "a bit under the weather" one or more times a month. That's a lot of folks. And, potentially, a lot of referrals.

More and more, pharmacists are seeing an opportunity—professional as well as financial—to play a more active role in diagnosing and minimally treating individuals for relatively minor conditions. And, as important, pharmacists are increasingly being seen as vital players in the treatment process for such activities as monitoring patient progress, educating the patient, and referring the patient to other services.

The Pharmacist's Increasing Role in Self-Care

Today, pharmacists have a small but effective arsenal of diagnostic tools at their disposal right in the store. In addition to the traditional monitoring devices for blood pressure and glucose, home test kits are becoming more available. The home test kit is by itself a vital force in the healthcare market. Coupled with the knowledge of a professional, it becomes a source of power.

Let's look at the dynamics of the home test market and its potential effect on the IDN.

The self-care market appears to be robust. *Drug Topics*, September 5, 1994, projected that home testing and diagnostics alone will be a $3.9 billion industry by the year 2000, nearly triple the 1993 level. That calculates out to an 18 percent compounded annual growth rate. The important indicator here is not so much that the sales volume will increase, but that the corresponding use rates will increase. Higher consumption of these types of tests and devices can create opportunities for referrals if properly directed.

Pregnancy tests are a case in point. According to A. C. Nielsen, a national consumer research company, 40 percent of women between the ages of 18 and 34 use pregnancy tests at least once a year (*Drug Topics*, August 19, 1996). Ninety percent report using the test at some point in their lives. Admittedly pregnancy is a unique example, but imagine the effect if the experience rate for pregnancy self-testing were repeated at just one-quarter of those levels among all product categories for all conditions. That scenario is becoming more and more feasible, given our increasingly educated, self-reliant population.

Traditionally viewed as an activity for blood glucose monitoring at home, home testing and its market are broadening their base in three basic directions: screening, diagnosis, and monitoring. The distinctions are important.

The screening and diagnostic categories are the two most rapidly expanding segments. Once characterized by pregnancy tests, the category now expects strong growth in areas such as home testing for HIV, urinary tract infection, strep throat, and other conditions.

Advances in biological and other technologies are certain to add applications beyond the areas now addressed.

A self-test takes on an added dimension of credibility and, most likely, accuracy when recommended and reviewed by a health professional such as a pharmacist. Repeated studies have shown that pharmacists have considerable credibility among consumers, and their recommendations are widely heeded.

A Profession in Search of Support

Right now, the pharmacist's chief clinical partner appears to be the pharmaceutical industry. The activity focuses on influencing the pharmacists' recommendations for self-choice items, or items in which the consumer can be "switched" to another product of equal efficacy. Marketing budgets among manufacturers have shifted dramatically over the past few years in recognition of the role pharmacists play in creating "instant" referrals. IDNs may want to consider the same move.

In fact, the smart money says an aggressive IDN may want to seek partnership with *both* the pharmaceutical manufacturer and the retailer to extend marketing dollars and create a more complete clinical loop.

The Threat

The initial threat, of course, is that the IDN is left of out of the picture altogether. And right now that appears to be exactly what's happening.

For example, the pharmacist builds a relationship with consumers and directs them according to his or her best judgment. Translation: the referrals are going just about anywhere. The IDN should seek control of those referrals.

Add to that activity the emergence of "pharmaceutical care." As the magazine *Drug Topics* reported in its August 5, 1996, issue, "Pharmacists know their profession is becoming more focused on patient care. But as they grow from drug dispensers to drug information resources, they often need help implementing a clinical practice and getting paid for their expanded role. Pharmaceutical care models help provide their assistance."

I hope you caught the key phrase "implementing a clinical practice." What does that mean? That pharmacists will be competing with physicians as care providers? Repeating the managed care mantra—"most appropriate care at the lowest-cost site"—rivets our attention. Indeed, the pharmacist may be the newest leg on the care delivery model.

Pharmacists themselves admit that an exact definition and role of pharmaceutical care is elusive at this point. But given the sheer economic incentives of survival, it is clearly more than a hula hoop trend. Indeed, American Druggist's "Survey of Pharmaceutical Care" reports that 54.3 percent of all retail pharmacists have begun practicing this service. And according to a comprehensive study by Find/SVP, New York, "Concept Pharmacy: What Is Pharmaceutical Care?" the results on patient outcomes is measurable. Some examples include:

- Emergency department visits for a group of 25 asthma patients was reduced to 6 from 47.
- A savings of $2,118 (1985 dollars) when anticoagulation patients are monitored by pharmacists.
- A savings of $377 per inpatient admission when a pharmacist is added to the team.

A New Beachhead for Managed Care

As MCOs continue to push care to the lowest-cost site possible, pharmacies become more attractive. They are widely distributed. They have a full-time healthcare professional who is not salaried by the MCO. And pharmacists are looking for what the MCO has a lot of—members who will become traffic in their stores.

It shouldn't come as a surprise that MCOs are beginning to use these sites. United Healthcare in Minneapolis is one of several MCOs using pharmacies to dispense adult flu shots for members. It's a natural.

Once MCOs connect the diagnostic capabilities of pharmacists with the first-line treatment of over-the-counter medications (OTCs), a new level of care will be initiated. Once again, it will be at the expense of the providers.

An Early Overture

The Walgreens stores in Chicago ran an interesting promotion in spring 1997. They essentially got into the diagnostics business by offering screenings for osteoporosis. And at a very attractive price of $29.95. According to the company, over 6,000 Chicago-area women took advantage of the offer.

A Walgreens's spokesperson says that the program is one of several screening efforts the chain has conducted across the country. In addition to osteoporosis, the stores have screened 4,000 men in Tampa, Florida for prostate cancer, plus several thousand in Chicago for colorectal cancer.

Walgreens indicates that it "likes" these programs for three primary reasons:

1. They raise community awareness about diseases.
2. Community involvement enhances Walgreens's image.
3. The programs bring added traffic through the store.

Walgreens believes that by identifying individuals with health problems, it creates long-term loyalty. "Consumers seem to like and want these programs," said a spokesperson at Walgreens. "Based on what we've seen, we will probably continue to look at different types of screenings."

With more than 2,300 stores in 36 states, Walgreens is a provider. A competitor.

The Opportunities

By their own admission, pharmacists are struggling to find a clear path to increasing their role both clinically and financially in the care of the patient. IDNs, with their geographic spread and resident knowledge, represent an ideal business partner for the pharmacist. Here's how.

Become an Educational Resource

The pharmacist's increasing role in early diagnosis of more and more health problems creates the need for more education and training. While pharmaceutical manufacturers can play a role in this regard, they will of course focus on those areas with the highest return. The IDN can take a higher road by addressing a broader number of clinical issues and presenting a complete course of care as opposed to a purely medical solution. The expectation is that the relationship will result in a higher number of referrals to the IDN.

Teaching hospitals are probably already implementing these types of programs. Such programs simply need to be leveraged to the marketing advantage of the IDN.

Create Retail Events

Retailers thrive on traffic—the grand march of consumers through their doors. The higher the traffic, the higher the sales. IDNs are seeking new ways to meet individuals and bring them into their systems. A logical step is to use the retailer as a site for any number of health-related events from screenings to other activities. Both benefit in sales and referrals. Both use their key resources—distribution from the retailer and knowledge from the provider.

Establish a Referral Network

If pharmacists are making referrals for dozens of consumers a day, *make your IDN the recipient of that business.* A referral network for pharmacists isn't much different from the one for referring physicians. A pharmacy program can be created for referrals just like the program you have in place right now for physicians and consumers.

Leverage Your National Alliance

For better or worse, the retail pharmacy business is now a national business. According to *Drug Store News*, May 19, 1997,

"State of the Industry Report" 45 percent (17,671 stores), of retail pharmacies are now part of national and regional chains.

National alliances can play an important role in creating relationships with these chains by offering the distribution of their members and the volume of their patient base. The IDNs can offer clinical resources and other programs in exchange for referrals.

This is just a smattering of ideas to move on in coming to terms with a dynamically emerging and strategically important player. Move fast and seize the opportunity.

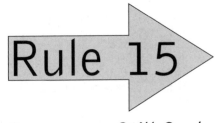

Rule 15

Consumers Still Seek Solutions to Their Health Problems

Something must have snapped in the minds of some decision makers when they reorganized into health-care systems. Somehow, they thought, this "system thing" will give us new relevance to people. So they abandoned their traditional and customarily successful approach of presenting solutions to healthcare problems and replaced it with a more corporate message. There is reason to believe the new approach isn't sticking.

One of the major attractions of healthcare in the consumer market has been its ability to solve a wide range of problems. Neither IDNs nor anyone else in the business can afford to abandon that strategy.

Product Lines Revisited

Product-line marketing is an example of what I call the "problem-solution" equation. The translation is pretty straightforward: show how you can solve a consumer's health problem.

But products were more narrowly defined when the emphasis was on the hospital-based product line. The products usually focused on a hospital-based solution. And the appeal proved to be limited given the course of treatment (the "inconvenience" of hospitalization) and the high cost.

Now is the time to give product lines new life, with new appeal.

If you can change your IDN marketing frame of reference from a "collection of properties" to a "deep resource of solutions," you may have the key to greater success in the market.

Executives agree that an "integrated" solution is the goal, but that it's a dream still on the horizon. At this point, it's probably best to link prevention to treatment to aftercare, for example, later on in the development of the product. Right now, solutions can be simpler.

By keeping breadth of solutions in mind, your IDN can have market appeal without having to impose a singular response (meaning hospitals)—and without moving to *too* much breadth before you're ready to back up your claims.

A large teaching hospital in the Midwest is a case in point. Looking for a way to leverage both teaching expertise and clinical skills, the hospital chose a road less traveled. Rather than competing with other medical centers over the traditional cardiology/oncology issues, they broke through the clutter with a direct assault on stomach disorders.

What's important about the effort is how effectively they positioned themselves not just for routine problems, but for the more severe (and appropriate) cases. Their advertising spoke to the patient who was frustrated with current unsuccessful treatments by citing their doctors' effectiveness in discovering and administering many new treatments for these chronic problems.

The marketing staff developed with their physicians a very clever telephone assessment tool that screened callers and immediately scheduled appointments for those who were in need. With a limited budget and modest use of print and radio, the effort generated over 800 appointments.

In its November 1997 report "Future Sources of Revenue: Sustainable Growth Strategies for America's Health Systems," The Health Care Advisory Board, Washington, D.C., compared the advertising efforts of large Midwestern health systems. One used a branding approach and the other spoke of specific expertise in heart and cancer. According to the analysis, the branding approach created a greater number of calls, but the problem-solution approach yielded a 128 percent higher appointment for rate services. Further analysis showed that of the calls for the problem-solution approach, 63 percent were for specialists, versus only 40 percent in the branded approach.

The example is not to trash branded advertising. It is an essential element to the overall effort. But the numbers do illustrate the difference between establishing a brand and, in effect, asking for the order.

Marketers need to expand their arsenal of solutions to health problems. In mature markets, hospitals are dying products. Many are hanging on to them because of their economic legacy, not their economic future. Alternative medicine, home care, self-testing, telephone counseling, and other innovations—solutions being demanded by the marketplace—can be added to the mix. Understanding exactly how each step of the way relates to the next can come at a later date.

Today, IDNs need to offer a combination of convenience, expertise, and service. We've entered a market of people who are much more curious, involved, and demanding than they used to be. The IDN, more than any other organization, should be able to respond to the needs of these new consumers by aggregating its vast resources to do what it does best—solve problems.

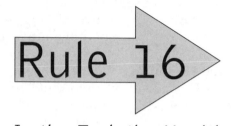

Rule 16

In the End, the Healthcare Choice Is Still an Emotional Decision

Wouldn't it be great if the world made all of its decisions rationally? Maybe so, but it's a moot point. We're not a terribly rational society when we purchase things, especially healthcare.

More and more providers are being forced into making a business argument on why they should be selected. And in the wholesale market, that indeed is the way decisions are made. It gets you on the short list of providers from which employees choose.

But in the retail market, where the final selection of a provider is made, healthcare choices, like thousands of other purchasing decisions, are based on emotion—not logic.

America Buys on Emotion

Look at the ways that many of the major brands in America communicate. Whether it's an airline, a tire company, or a fast food chain, it's using emotion as the glue that bonds us to the brand.

- United Airlines shows us how responsive it is.

- Michelin Tires suggests that its product is the best protection on the road for our families.

- Wendy's hamburgers are served by their smiling CEO just to show us how down home they really are.

The list of examples is endless. All of these brands use emotion as the basis for the bond. They support their messages with the traditional features and benefits of on-time service, price promotion, and the rest. But their branded message has a strong emotional appeal. These marketers understand that "the facts" are persuasive only to a point—that in the end, a service brand without an emotional link to its customers underperforms in the category.

If you identify with the mindset of today's healthcare customer, you'll find yourself confused, frustrated, and perhaps even angry. Will a rational argument about your capabilities create a bond with your brand? Can fact after fact about your clinical performance and medical credentials tilt the needle in your direction if you are seen as an uncaring place? Most likely not. The results from the Press, Ganey, Kaiser Foundation, and other studies conclude that, no, it won't.

Another in a continuing series of studies is "Eye on Patients: A Report to the American Public," conducted in 1996 by the Picker Institute, a Boston-based health consumer research firm. The report indicates that in the area of staff courtesy and hotel services, only 4 to 7 percent of those surveyed gave their doctors, nurses, or other staff low ratings for basic courtesy. In fact, patients found their surroundings to be generally comfortable. But they "felt that care givers did not provide emotional support as they went through their procedures or treatment." And, the report continued, "patients describe a feeling of being abandoned when they are released from the hospital—like jumping off into nowhere." The Harvard and University of Kansas study mentioned earlier bears the statistical proof to this claim.

Psychologists tell us that it's not just "health" we're talking about in discussing healthcare. The subject is emotionally far reaching and touches our relationships with others. A health problem represents a relationship crisis with those we know or love. It threatens to change the relationship. Unalterably. Forever. No hospital performance fact in the world will alleviate the reality of that fear, that stunning awareness that the future may be different.

Do providers recognize that? More important, are they able to communicate to their customers that they empathize, that they can be a source of support?

A Product Not a Promotional Strategy

Empathy is not a promotional strategy. It must be part of the product. Marketing's job is to make sure that element of the product—empathy—is in place and recognized by the end users and by those who influence the product's purchase.

The Kaiser study showed that at least for now consumers are more likely to be influenced by qualitative information, not quantitative. Translation: it's emotional truth, not statistical fact, that makes the compelling argument.

Healthcare is arguably the most emotional industry in America. It has to be. Health determines the quality of our life, our ability to earn an income, our chances to pursue our dreams. Can anyone expect to influence those expectations through fact and logic?

Not entirely.

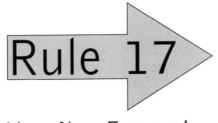

Rule 17

Your New Economic Frame of Reference Is Called "PMPM"

As we all know, economics is as much a fact of life as health, and our wholesale and retail customers must deal with the logic of their enterprises—their facts and figures. An integrated delivery network has to balance economics and healthcare, and the balance is a precarious one.

If you want to understand your wholesale customer's motivation, you need to understand its economic drivers. For hospitals it used to be revenue, contribution to margin, profitability, or some other indicator. With the exception of profitability, MCOs look at the world from a totally different perspective.

As we all know, too, capitation gives the plan a set amount each month for each member. The acronym is "PMPM," which translates into "per member per month." The translation for a provider is simple: "I've only got this amount of money to take care of this individual. Any expense I deduct from this amount directly affects my profitability. I am given the incentive to not spend money."

According to Hoechst Marion Roussel's 1996 *Managed Care Digest*, the average monthly revenue per member for HMOs was slightly over $118. Taking this figure as an example (it may or may not be accurate by the time you read this), most plans try to target 85 percent of those dollars to cover medical costs with the remainder split between administration and profit. So, of the $118, approximately $100.30 per month goes for patient care and $17.70 for administration and profit. As you try to add value or negotiate better rates, understand that a cost of as little as five cents PMPM can be a deal breaker.

Managed care organizations use a PMPM calculation in their budgets for marketing activities. The range of marketing expense can range significantly, a factor usually associated with the stage of market development of the plan. In one start-up HMO with 60,000 members we are working with, marketing costs are budgeted at $1.04 PMPM. Just across the state, an established HMO with 600,000 members budgets around $0.11 PMPM.

Using a Value-Based Approach

Similarly, when you try to create value with a payor, your value-added programs might make a greater value statement if they are expressed as savings for the MCO. For example, if one of your value-added programs is assistance with HEDIS compliance, that activity could translate into a PMPM savings. For example, screenings, one of HEDIS's more costly requirements, can easily be translated in a cost either per member or PMPM that the IDN is absorbing in exchange for a broader base of business. It may not be enough to cinch a deal, but at least you'll be negotiating in terms that the payor understands and in an area that is critical to the plan's success.

In the art of negotiation, one of the basic rules is to play back strategies that your opponent uses against you. In this case, your "high cost" may be converted into a PMPM savings.

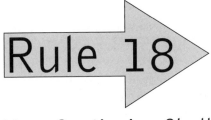

Rule 18

Your Continuing Challenge to Succeed Is Your Ability to Gain and Sustain Focus

"Dear Mr. Sturm, We are out of Pepsi and the vacuum caught on fire."

—Mary, my former cleaning lady

It's pretty clear from that note that Mary has her priorities straight. Part of her terms of employment were that I keep a supply of Pepsi® at her disposal. The fact that the vacuum caught on fire (and fortunately not the rest of the place) was secondary. Mary had focus. She was single-minded and knew her priorities.

Open your desk drawer and pull out your list of strategic initiatives for the year. Count them up. My guess is that there are a lot of them, most likely in the range of a dozen or so well-intentioned efforts that need to be addressed.

How realistic is it to hope that all of these initiatives will succeed? Not very. At a time when resources are scarce and demands are high, success suffers. Focus, unfortunately, is not always a popular concept in executive offices. But it has to be for the marketer.

The Rule of Two

The concept of focus for the marketer might easily be interchanged with that of "sacrifice." To keep your focus in today's tug-of-war of ideas you have to decide what can be sacrificed to make sure the key initiatives succeed. It's not easy. "Sacrifice is the essence of strategy," said David Ogilvy, one of marketing's great brand builders.

On a more practical level, I always work with the Rule of Two. The Rule of Two says you can have as many strategic initiatives as you like, as long as it's not more than two. That may sound rather smug, but experience has taught me that the more focused efforts greatly outperform the scattered ones.

Focus supports my basic belief that in marketing you need to "own" something. Ownership translates into dominance in a category or segment. When you gear up to own something, you direct all of the resources necessary not just to compete but to dominate. You most likely won't have the resources to own more than two of anything, but if you dilute those same resources against several fronts, you are likely to own nothing.

The Singular Focus of Your Brand

The challenge becomes particularly critical—as well as difficult—in developing a brand for the IDN. The temptation, by nature, is to say everything possible about all of the benefits your IDN has to offer. But doing so is a sure step to failure.

People don't want to know everything about your IDN. They want simply to find out about something relevant to them, their families, and their lives. A grocery list of services doesn't meet that need.

But we've discussed the idea of singularity in other chapters. Here the admonition is to *sustain that singularity* as well as create it. The challenges to change direction are going to be relentless. How many well-meaning board members, physicians, administrators, and colleagues will say, "Hey, I think we ought to be saying. . . ." Let's not bother to count.

While many of their ideas probably have merit, the truth is that the strategy train has already set out on its course. It has left the station. The more you change directions and messages, the longer it will take you to get anywhere in the mind of the target, be it consumer, payor, employer, or board member.

Sustaining the Focus

One behavior that has always surprised me about health-care is its constant movement from one initiative to another before it has maximized the benefit of the first. I call this the "butterfly strategy," recalling how in spring the butterfly flits from flower to flower. That's nice to do if you are only going to be around for a little while (butterflies only live for a few weeks), but it's not recommended for organizations that want a longer lifespan (we're hoping for decades, not days).

Marketing thrives on consistency. That means it may get a little boring to the folks on the inside, but a constantly reinforced brand message sticks in the mind of the market. For instance, Volvo has been running its safety positioning since the 1960s. Over that period its sales have grown, and its share has expanded. Volvo's brand managers have been able to keep the idea of safety fresh in the minds of people through strong advertising that never sways from the brand's position.

Volvo has been extremely creative in keeping a rather dull idea fresh, memorable, and singular. Consistency does not automatically default into boredom.

You should commit yourself to an equally strict discipline of focus. And stick with it.

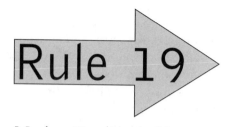

Rule 19

Make Radical Changes in the Organizational Structure of Your Marketing Department

Historically, provider marketing has had mixed results in organizing around product-line models. There was a cardiology group, a cancer group, and a physician relations group. Sales fit in there somewhere. In the new world of healthcare marketing, a more radical approach may be beneficial.

American Express (Amex) learned that a radical approach paid off. Until 1992 it used traditional product-line marketing. It had a Gold Card marketing department, as well as one for Optima, one for Platinum, and still another for the Green Card (called "The Personal Card" by Amex).

Amex learned that this approach was just too unorganized. Because each group ran its own program, they often found themselves in competition. They were often operating in conflict with other cards, thus reducing results overall for the parent.

The company finally came to the conclusion that it had to move away from selling individual products and start managing individual customers and customer relationships. To do this, it had to come up with a total restructuring of

card-marketing operations. Managers were held accountable for a share of customer objectives rather than for product sales. Their charge—to implement strategies based on
service quality and loyalty.

If in the new world healthcare customers are going to
be either members or nonmembers, perhaps your marketing
department should be organized accordingly. Not so much
around the idea of members and nonmembers, but under
the more proactive banners of "acquisition and retention."

Their respective roles seem pretty clear.

The Acquisition Group

This team functions on two levels: contracting and enrollment. It seems logical and important that the two efforts
work side by side. The enrollment folks need to know what's
in the contract. They can be a resource to the contracting
agent by providing feedback on what new members are
responding to most. And they can talk about changes they
are making to improve member satisfaction.

By moving contracting out of finance and into marketing, IDNs have a greater opportunity to enter a more seamless negotiation. Because value propositions can be more
easily explored and developed between the acquisition and
retention teams, they can be brought to the bargaining table
full grown, the defenses in place, ready for approval.

The acquisition group is the keeper of the brand, the
tracker of market trends, the manager of sales and relationships with wholesalers, brokers, and employers. The job of
acquisitions is to make a seamless transfer of a new member
into the programs of the retention group.

The Retention Group

The charge here is obvious:

- to keep members;
- to find ways to measure, track, and improve member satisfaction;
- to find ways to create additional revenue streams from members; and
- to integrate the retention group into the operations of the member facilities.

The retention group is the advocate of the member. By tracking member needs through research and database monitoring, the retention group is responsible for getting operations to respond to customer needs. Higher response rates lead to higher satisfaction resulting, one hopes, in stronger retention.

Other Roles Become Critical Support Elements

So what happens to the traditional departments of research, public relations, and advertising? Frankly, not much, except that they now have a clearer context in which to work. In Figure 19.1, these traditional areas become resources to

Figure 19.1 The New Marketing Organization

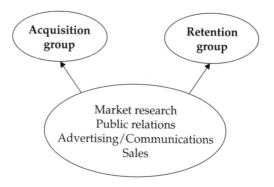

the key initiative, much as they always have been. They are responsible under this model for supporting the key strategic initiatives of acquisition and retention.

With this acquisition and retention model, goals and incentives can be more clearly aligned, and senior management can see an organizational structure that complements a larger corporate initiative.

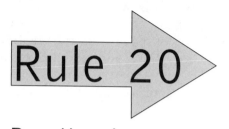

Rule 20

Be a Hero in a Tumultuous Market

"59 percent of Americans surveyed favor national health insurance."
—The Wirthkin Report, November, 1996

"Overall, participants felt there was no one in the healthcare field advocating for them."
—from a report in AHA News (December 16, 1996) on consumer issues facing providers.

Healthcare has lost its halo. Time was when medical breakthroughs were received with great awe and enthusiasm. Now they are greeted with "it's about time." It seems like a no-win situation for providers.

Today's tumultuous market represents some opportunities for providers to demonstrate a real interest in the health and well-being of their customers. Legislative challenges to HMOs is a case in point. With managed care moving to reduce hospital stays rather dramatically, the market is looking for "heroes." Might as well be you.

How do you become a hero? The marketplace makes it easy.

Providers are drawing a negative response from consumers because of their constant public debates on cost and profits. The marketplace evidently doesn't care too much for the scent of money. As a study by the Kaiser Family Foundation showed in 1997, 47 percent of the Americans surveyed think "for profit" healthcare is "a bad thing."

A Starting Point: Create a New Category of Organizations

Research has shown that the term "not-for-profit organization" has become meaningless to the American public. Once hospitals were seen as organizations that were not motivated by profit. But given their current size and economics it has proved difficult for consumers to apply the term "not-for-profit" and feel comfortable with it.

Private sector hospitals long ago realized that there was not much value in being referred to as "for-profit" hospitals. So they created a seemingly new category for themselves called "investor owned." Similarly, the pharmaceutical industry found that if it talked about its research mission, consumers were more understanding of their pricing. And so they positioned themselves as research companies, not just as manufacturers. Not-for-profit hospitals need to make the same adjustment.

The challenge now is to create this category for IDNs. One term that is being used that deserves further support is "community benefit organization." The idea is being pioneered by BJC Health System in St. Louis, Missouri.

On first blush, the term at least sounds like it's moving in the right direction. It needs greater substance to be lasting and effective. But it, or a similar concept, deserves exploration.

Heroes and Heroines

The healthcare debate is creating more than rancor—it's creating confusion. Someone could be a hero to the consumer by directing some dollars into explaining—and reinforcing—what the changes mean. The list of topics is endless. Start with new legislation on portability of benefits and move to a basic primer on managed care.

And the legislative arena provides another opportunity for heroes. Witness those smart organizations that responded to managed care's "drive-through deliveries" initiatives with a pledge that the moms could stay the second night free. Consumers felt that the hospital had stood up for them. They had an advocate; someone was fighting for them. A hero was at work.

Three Ideas to Pursue

Here are three basic opportunities that IDNs might consider to reverse their downward impression in local markets.

1. Stand for Something

In the debate over the future of healthcare, providers seem to be noticeably absent. Admittedly, they have had a quiet voice in the past, but today there is too much attention directed at healthcare to assume that it can quietly sidestep the limelight.

Standing for something is a vast oversimplification for a strategy that says the IDN needs to be recognized for a particular point of view and to be adamant in its pursuit. There is no shortage of issues on which to take a stand. Choose one and work to own it.

2. Be a Voice of Reason

Earlier I talked about the need to reposition healthcare organizations as something called "community benefit organizations." One thing that would benefit communities greatly would be a reasoned voice, someone who could present the issues fairly and clearly with the appearance of the least amount of self-interest.

In chapter 16, I talk about healthcare being an emotional decision. It is also an emotional topic. People tend to go ballistic just at the mention of the word. Doesn't it seem like the leadership thing to do to offer a more balanced perspective on the issues?

While providers' credibility has been challenged, it has not been totally erased. Serving as the voice of reason on issues may be a key way to enhance the IDN as well as the industry.

3. Be an Interpreter

The healthcare polemic needs an interpreter. If, as research has shown, most people don't understand healthcare's basic vocabulary, how can the industry expect the market to understand its issues? Seems unlikely.

There is a tremendous need—and a corresponding opportunity—to help consumers understand the issues and the many consequences of change. Some IDNs have begun working on this need, but the information has been confined to company-sponsored publications. Broader, more persistent communication is necessary to reach the vast and growing populations that IDNs serve.

As an emerging industry, IDNs have a window of opportunity to recast public opinion of the healthcare delivery system. But, like other windows, it will be open just until "the wind starts blowing." The cost of passage is low compared with the expense of undoing greater confusion in the future.

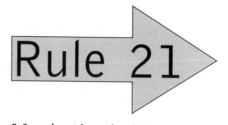

Rule 21

Marketing's New Accountability Is the 4 Rs

That's not a typo It's now the 4 Rs, not the 4 Ps (product, price, place, and promotion) that many of us grew up with.

The four Rs are recruitment, retention, referrals, and return. Let's look at each one.

Recruitment

Historically, healthcare has looked at recruitment as an employee issue. But in a managed care environment, the goal is to recruit or attract members. Marketing's principal responsibility is to see that contracts are maximized for the greatest pull-through of members. Other chapters of this book have identified strategies for recruitment. The important lesson here is to integrate a membership goal into the performance measures of the marketing department.

Retention

Logic rules here. If we spend a considerable amount of resources getting members, we should be equally concerned with keeping them from year to year. While actual numbers may vary, many industry experts believe that for every five dollars you spend to get a new member, it only takes one dollar to retain them. In the Saturn example mentioned earlier, only 5 percent of its advertising dollars were spent on retention, but the retained customers netted 50 percent of the dealer's revenues.

The role of marketing in retention should be significant. It starts by measuring member satisfaction and then having the ability to work with operations to see that those scores improve.

Retention, of course, requires a lot more than measuring satisfaction. It is a proactive strategy whereby the IDN makes conscious efforts to secure the renewal of those individual commitments to the system. Retention programs can take many forms in many venues. It is first a philosophy that must pervade the system. "Bring 'em back" has to be a continuing theme that runs through each facility, each department, every internal communication, every action.

Marketing must also find ways for the organization to create value—significant, differentiating value—for the membership. As noted earlier, the marketplace's expectations continually rise. Creating value is no small task, but it is one that must be thoughtfully done and repeated often. Each market defines value uniquely and the IDN must respond to those particular needs.

Referrals

If vast sums of money and energy have been used to create an IDN, an obvious and inherent need is to see that all units have sufficient business to survive. An earlier marketing idea held that the system would generate enough internal referrals to keep the various businesses going. But with the emerging consumer market, opportunities exist to capture transient demand and direct it to the entities of the IDN. It's marketing's job to see that that gets done.

As IDNs move away from hospitals, the need for a central ability to capture and direct referrals to other healthcare services becomes critical. Whether it's with nursing homes, health clubs, or chiropractic services, the integrated system must have an efficient means of matching its services to the needs of the community. It's not likely that advertising dollars will amount to enough to support each entity, but if the brand is positioned as a broad provider of services, the network should be able to capture and distribute demand accordingly.

Banks have demonstrated that they can build a brand as a financial service center; they now direct the market to a wide range of services from banking to brokerage to insurance. The same opportunity exists for IDNs, and it's marketing's responsibility to stimulate and channel that demand.

Return

Return on investment is not a new concept for healthcare marketers. It has just become a more compelling one. Many not-for-profit IDNs struggle with what constitutes an acceptable rate of return for their organizations. Whatever number works for your organization is an individual matter to pursue. But pursue it you must, and hold marketing accountable for it.

One note of caution. Return must be measured in actual dollars, over a specified time period. And in the latter element, some considerations need to be made. Building a new IDN and changing the behavior of the marketplace is never an overnight effort. If you move a large contract your way, obviously the return is quick. But if you are moving a larger share of the market to nonhospital services, the effort may take longer.

In creating strategic and marketing plans for your organization, consider aligning the goals and incentives to measurements that are most likely to ensure success.

Rule 22

In an Impersonal World, Find the Right Handshake

First impressions mean a lot in our society. Many of us form lasting impressions based on nothing more than a handshake. It is no different for an institution than it is for a person. Handshakes make a difference.

Retailer Wal-Mart demonstrated the importance of this simple act. By using a greeter at each of their stores they immediately reframed the shopping experience from an impersonal trek through the aisles to a more personable enjoyable part of the day. Today, hundreds of other retailers emulate this strategy to make customers feel more relaxed and a little more at home in an unfamiliar environment.

For years, healthcare providers relied on the first encounter at the hospital as their handshake. But if you think about it, that moment is probably a little too late. Given an IDN's diversity and the efforts to keep consumers away from hospitals, it seems clear that a handshake needs to happen in other places and in other ways. Here's a look at a few that can be critical moments in your ability to begin a positive experience and a loyal relationship.

Your call center

The smart IDN will realize the growing importance of the call center both as a handshake and as a core marketing service. Call centers—through their ability to create referrals to physicians and services, register consumers for classes or dispense healthcare information—more and more are becoming the first point of contact between the users and the provider.

If you want to find out how this handshake works for you, call it. See how long it takes to have your call answered. Ask yourself if that call helped you feel more positive about the sponsor. Did the call center try to help you build a relationship by referring you to one of their sites, suggest a class or program even if you didn't ask for one, and admit that they couldn't help you but referred you to someone who could?

The experience was a handshake. A sort of telephonic "howdy." If it was limp and impersonal, you essentially begged the caller to go somewhere else the next time.

Your Advertising

As advertising becomes more prominent, its role becomes more valuable. Susan Gillette, former president of Chicago-based DDB Needham, a major consumer advertising agency, often referred to advertising as a product's handshake to the market. "It often time is the first exposure the market has to your brand," she said, "and if it is cold and impersonal, confusing, or otherwise unfriendly, you've probably lost an opportunity."

Remember this when looking at your positioning work. Are you putting so much emphasis on talking about yourself that you inadvertently blow off a potential relationship?

In the world of packaged goods, marketers are always trying to give consumers the opportunity to sample their products as a way to induce trial. We've all been offered freebies in the grocery store, the train station, or on street corners. It's done because it works. It's a handshake.

Providers have been using educational programs and screenings for years as a way for people to sample their organization. Maybe they should also look at it as a handshake.

Educational programs of all types have demonstrated their ability to draw people into an organization. They have been used as a means to profile physicians and other healthcare professionals and their expertise. Their value is often related to their link to the provider's mission. But on a different scale they represent a tangible, first-time experience with an unknown organization or individual. They can create a true and lasting impression, and begin an even more important relationship.

Your Web Site

Enough has been said about the emerging role of the Internet in healthcare. But if you are still looking for a perspective of where it fits in, try the handshake. And visit your own Web site to see just what type of first impression your making. Where's the emphasis? If it is all about your organization written in the "I-We" person, it's probably a pretty impersonal handshake.

There are plenty of other places to look for handshakes. In your doctor's offices, through your external publications and in any of the other ways that meet the public, find a way to let the personality of the brand come through.

The handshake isn't the most strategically significant thing you will ever do. But in an increasingly impersonal world, it's a key element in building a lasting relationship.

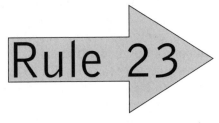

Rule 23

Learn from the Marketing Lessons of *Titanic*

When I went to summer camp as a kid, we used to sit around the campfire and sing folklore tales. One of them, of course, was about the great ocean liner *Titanic* ("and they thought they had a ship that the water couldn't get through") and very inaccurately recalled the history of that great tragedy. No wonder I went through most of my life convinced that on that fateful April night, a giant iceberg lurched from the floor of the Atlantic Ocean, grabbed the behemoth ship in its jaws, and savagely wrestled it to the bottom.

Although *Titanic* has recently been popularized in every entertainment medium known to man (including a Broadway musical), for many years I have characterized it as truly a lesson in marketing and management gone awry. There's no corn here about "healthcare being on a great voyage," but, instead, a true lesson in management. Market dynamics forced the development of *Titanic*, and bad management caused her demise. *Titanic*, like IDNs, represented a new approach to a well-entrenched behavior (transatlantic passage), but was so poorly managed that it almost killed an entire industry.

Titanic was one of two luxury cruise ships built by White Star Lines to help the company compete effectively in transatlantic transportation. Its competitor, Cunard Lines, had a ship that could cross the ocean in just five days. Unless White Star came up with a response, it would be at a significant competitive disadvantage.

White Star's strategy was to build a ship that was the ultimate in luxury and comfort. Speed, which caused a discomforting vibration on board, was sacrificed for a clearer point of difference—luxury.

Thus was *Titanic* born.

The analogy between an ocean liner and an IDN may seem impossible. And it is. But a somewhat closer parallel can be drawn by considering how bad decision making against a relatively sound business strategy can result in failure. Draw your own conclusions, but do so relative to the specifics of decision making. For they indeed are universal.

What Killed *Titanic*

Actually, three key management behaviors doomed the ship. Arrogance. Poor use of technology. And poor decision making. Here's how it happened.

Arrogance

It is somewhat common knowledge that *Titanic* lacked a sufficient number of lifeboats for passengers and crew. But it's the trail of that decision-making process that is most disturbing.

The British Board of Trade, the official agency governing vessels such as *Titanic*, somehow calculated that the ship needed only enough lifeboats for 962 lives. White Star, in some other form of delusion, thought that number too lenient and upped it to 1,178. With a full complement of crew and passengers, *Titanic* could accommodate 3,511 lives.

How could the ship's owners and the government oversight agency believe that the ship simply couldn't go down ever, under any circumstance? Watertight doors, said the owners, made her "practically unsinkable."

Historians view it differently. They see the error as one of arrogance. The owners as well as the regulators failed to acknowledge that *all ventures have a limit*. Regardless of the vision. Exclusive of resources. IDNs are not excluded from these rules.

Poor Use of Technology

In 1911, the hot new technology was the Marconi Wireless, a venture of the Marconi International Marine Communications Company, London. It was at that time a completely commercial venture offering passengers the novel opportunity to send missives to loved ones at home from sea. It was the cellular phone of the early 1900s.

Totally unregulated, the new instrument's role as a maritime and navigational aid was yet to come. It took a disaster to create the enabling legislation.

For days, *Titanic's* radio had been receiving word from other ships in the transatlantic shipping lanes of approaching heavy ice floes. But on April 14, the night of the collision, radio operator Jack Phillips was too involved in last-minute messages to find the time to take the life-saving warnings to the bridge. After all, he wasn't paid to do that.

Titanic sailed into the peril at full speed. It didn't have to.

Unfortunately, the problem compounded itself. Within four hours sail of *Titanic* was a potential rescue ship, the steamer *Carpathia*. Cyril Evans, *Carpathia's* radio operator, spent his evening eavesdropping on the personal messages of the soon-to-be-victims. Eventually bored, he turned off his listening device and retired at 11:35 p.m., less than two hours before *Titanic* sent her first wireless distress call. Had he continued to listen, he would have heard's *Titanic's* pleas; and a rescue might have been possible. Technology was poorly used.

IDNs are similarly challenged not just to seek out new technology, but to find a strong and productive role for it. The challenge is no longer the mere accumulation of technology, but its rightful distribution to serve the needs of the society that has enabled it to exist.

Bad Decision Making

John Smith was awarded the captaincy of *Titanic* because of his years of noble service to White Star. His career summary listed all of the important achievements befitting the captain of the world's largest ship.

But Smith abandoned his skills that night in April. He had received reports earlier in the day of increasing ice floes in the area. But he knew that if he continued at his present speed he could beat the record of *Titanic's* sister ship *Olympic* and gain yet another series of kudos for its sterling career. Aware of the potential danger but eager to succeed, he chose to leave the bridge early that night in the hands of younger, less experienced lieutenants. Smith's final orders were to maintain maximum speed in this, the final leg of the voyage.

Titanic, not having the advantages of normal sea trials, maneuvered much differently from other ships of the day. Her size made handling difficult. Inexperience made things worse.

When the officers on the bridge realized they were about to collide with an iceberg, First Officer Murdoch incorrectly reversed the engines. That action caused a slower turn away from the iceberg and made the collision inevitable. Had Murdoch simply turned away without reversing the engines, impact would likely have been avoided.

A bad decision indeed. But an even worse decision by the captain to leave an inexperienced crew to navigate perilous waters.

The analogies are many. IDNs by their size and clout in the market can easily slip into arrogance. The widespread availability of technology and the existing costs can create opportunities for abuse or misuse. And in the exuberance to succeed, bad decision making can proliferate.

Unfortunately, IDNs in the mind of the impatient public have had the luxury of sea trials. The market now expects the pursuit of a well-charted course and a reasonable sailing.

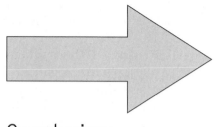

Conclusion:
Break the Rules

Marketing is one of those unique disciplines that behaves pretty much the way it wants to. In its purest form, it is driven by hard facts and tempered with emotion. It is replete with basic do's and don'ts, and it likes to think of itself as highly disciplined. Indeed it is. But it has also shown time and again that those who break the rules succeed.

Apple Computers did it when they launched the personal computer, Compaq Computers improved on their idea by offering a personal computer for under $1,000, and Oracle has created innovative database applications. These folks broke the rules of convention and succeeded—at least initially.

Over the past 20 years or so being part of the healthcare marketing phenomena, I've watched a lot of behaviors from boards on down. While the perspective of history is always educational, the new marketplace requires that we recast our thinking, our expectations, and even our definition of success. I've taken the liberty of identifying those behaviors that, at least in my view, will affect the likelihood of moving an organization forward.

One. Be passionate about your vision. "Visioning" has become so process driven, I wonder where the commitment comes in. It has to come from passion both in its development and in its execution. Without passion, marketing will be run solely by the numbers. There's too much emotion in the healthcare decision-making process to suggest a dispassionate strategy will prevail.

Two. Understand when to think inside and outside of the box. It seems marketing professionals are constantly being challenged to think "outside of the box." I think that's good, but they also need to be reminded of the need for balance. Often, traditional, tried-and-true strategies make sense. They do so because the competition hasn't tried them. Or they tried them and didn't execute them well. Or for any number of reasons. The tighter the market, the more you need to think outside of the box. Not on everything, but in those areas where you'll get the biggest return.

Three. Make physicians be marketing's biggest advocates. This is conclusion based on years of experience and observation. Marketing just doesn't work without strong physician participation. As difficult as they can be in development strategy, I haven't seen a program succeed yet without strong physician buy-in. And those programs have benefited greatly from a more passionate, committed physician group.

Four. Operationalize your brand strategy. I hope you realize by now that you don't have brand unless you behave like one. Most health system "marketing" that's out there consists of advertising to build name awareness. Branding will occur when you deliver some meaningful benefit day to day to your target audience. Once you get the physicians on board, get the operations people sitting with you, and get a commitment from your board, you can truly create a brand and not just an image.

Five. Avoid the "Butterfly Strategy." The butterfly strategy is an easy concept to grasp. Think about what butterflies do. They carefully select a target, land on it, then move quickly to another. And another. And another, never really staying very long. Healthcare seems to embrace the butterfly strategy more than I would like to see. If you agree that marketing thrives on consistency, then you have to be ruthless in support of it with your programs. Avoid at all costs the temptation to do all things for all people. In these times, your focus should be on the building the brand first and all other matters second.

The marketplace is rewriting all of the rules of healthcare everyday. From the delivery of care to the way it gets paid, the industry is constantly being challenged to reinvent itself.

If you are truly going to succeed in the marketplace, think of this book as you would computing technology. It's already out of date when you receive it, but it's got enough to it to get you through the next phase of market development.

Break the rules with better thinking, stronger leadership, and deeper commitments. And do it often.

About the Author

Arthur Sturm is president and CEO of Sturm Rosenberg King and Company, a Chicago-based healthcare marketing and advertising firm. Mr. Sturm is generally considered one of the nation's pioneers in healthcare marketing. Today he and his firm serve providers, pharmaceutical manufacturers, managed care organizations, healthcare consumer product companies, and others in the industry.

Mr. Sturm is widely published in trade magazines such as *Modern Healthcare*, *Medical Marketing and Media*, and *Advertising Age*. He is a frequent speaker and has appeared on national media including NBC, National Public Radio and others.

He is married and has two children who usually follow the rules.